8 SECRETS OF A

HEALTHY 100

| WHAT *do* YOU WANT *to* DO WHEN *you're* 100? |

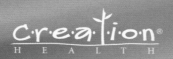

8 SECRETS OF A

HEALTHY

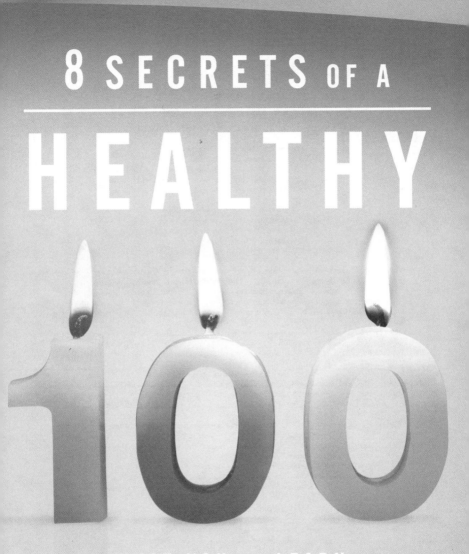

100

WHAT YOU CAN LEARN
FROM THE ALL-STARS OF LONGEVITY

DES CUMMINGS JR., PHD

with MONICA REED, MD and TODD CHOBOTAR

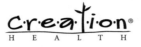

8 SECRETS OF A HEALHTY 100
Copyright © 2012 Des Cummings Jr.
Published by Florida Hospital Publishing
900 Winderley Place, Suite 1600, Maitland, FL 32751

TO EXTEND *the* HEALTH *and* HEALING MINISTRY *of* CHRIST

EDITOR-IN-CHIEF	Todd Chobotar
MANAGING EDITOR	David Biebel, DMin
PEER REVIEW	Eli Kim, MD, George Guthrie, MD
PEER REVIEW	Sy Saliba, PhD, Robyn Edgerton
PROMOTION	Laurel Dominesey
PRODUCTION	Lillian Boyd
COPY EDITOR	Pam Nordstrom
PHOTOGRAPHY	Spencer Freeman
COVER DESIGN	Studio Absolute
INTERIOR DESIGN	Retse Saylor
BUSINESS DEVELOPMENT	Stephanie Lind, MBA

PUBLISHER'S NOTE: This book is not intended to replace a one-on-one relationship with a qualified healthcare professional but as a sharing of knowledge and information from the research and experience of the author. You are advised and encouraged to consult with your healthcare professional in all matters relating to your health and the health of your family. The publisher and author disclaim any liability arising directly or indirectly from the use of this book.

AUTHOR'S NOTE: This book contains many case histories and patient stories. In order to preserve the privacy of some of the people involved, I have disguised names, appearances, and aspects of their personal stories so they are not identifiable. Patient stories may also include composite characters.

For volume discounts please contact special sales at:
HealthProducts@FLHosp.org | 407-303-1929

*Cataloging-in-Publication Data for this book
is available from the Library of Congress.
Printed in the United States of America.*
PR 14 13 12 11 10 9 8 7 6 5 4 3 2 1
ISBN 13: 978-0-9820409-1-1

For more Whole Person Health resources visit:
**FloridaHospitalPublishing.com
Healthy100Churches.org
CreationHealth.com
Healthy100.org**

CONTENTS

Foreword — Why the Adventists? 6

1. Go After Life
   The Spirit of a Healthy 100 8

2. Why Would I Want to Live to 100?
   Overcoming the Barriers to a Healthy 100 12

3. What You Can Learn from the All-Stars of Longevity
   Origin of the 8 Secrets 17

4. C — Choice
   First We Make Choices, Then Choices Make Us 27

5. R — Rest
   We Live with Stress, But We Don't Have to Die From It 41

6. E — Environment
   You Were Made for a Garden, But You Live in a Jungle 53

7. A — Activity
   How Activity Fuels Energy and Power-Filled Living 66

8. T — Trust
   Why Trust is the Most Powerful Health Tool of All 81

9. I — Interpersonal
   Love is Only Realized in Relationship 92

10. O — Outlook
    Pursuing the Positive Power of Optimism and Hope 105

11. N — Nutrition
    Feeding the Body, Nurturing the Mind, Inspiring the Spirit 119

12. Creating Your Family's Health Legacy
    Passing a Healthy Lifestyle from Generation to Generation 132

13. What Inspires You to Live?
    How Do You Plan to Live as Fully as Possible for as Long as Possible? 143

Acknowledgments 147

About the Authors 148

About the Publisher 150

Endnotes 151

Resources 155

FOREWORD

Why The Adventists?

I F I POSSESSED A PILL THAT COULD EXTEND LIFE
by eleven years it would be considered a wonder drug and would
be sought after by millions. I would feel obligated to make this pill
available to you, your family, and the world so that everyone could
enjoy the benefits of a longer, healthier life. While I do not have
such a pill, I do know a lifestyle that could add an average of eleven
years to your life. In many ways it's better than a pill because it has
no adverse side effects.

This lifestyle has been researched, documented, and verified
over the last fifty years. In a special edition of *National Geographic*
entitled "The Secrets of Living Longer," author Dan Buettner
highlighted three major lifestyles: Okanawans in Japan, Sardinians
in Italy, and Adventists in Loma Linda, California. This latter group
he identified as the *All-Stars of Longevity* in America. While all three
groups produce longevity all-stars, the Adventist lifestyle is unique
because it is the most universally transferable of the three.

It has been replicated in populations around the world.

It is not genetically dependent and can transfer across races and
ethnic groups.

It has produced more people who have reached one hundred years
of age than any other lifestyle in America—a remarkable achievement
in a culture moving in the opposite health direction today.

This research is increasingly being acknowledged in mainstream
media. For example, a *US News* report said, "Americans who define
themselves as Seventh-day Adventists have an average life expectancy
of 89, about a decade longer than the average American. One of the

basic tenets of the religion is that it's important to cherish the body that's on loan from God, which means no smoking, alcohol abuse, or overindulging in sweets. Followers typically stick to a vegetarian diet based on fruits, vegetables, beans, and nuts, and get plenty of exercise. They're also very focused on family and community."[1]

The Adventist health lifestyle was part of a "clean living" movement that emerged in America during the 1800s. Various groups led by health advocates promoted the value of fresh air, water, sunshine, exercise, and a plant-based diet. They also pointed out the health dangers of tobacco, drugs, alcohol, caffeine, and red meat. The Adventist leaders traced the origin of many of these practices to Scripture and encouraged church members to incorporate them into daily life. I share this with you so that you can have an understanding that these ideas were not exclusive to the Adventist church. They are concepts open for your examination, criticism, advancement, and adoption.

> No matter what your faith background or health history, this book was written for you.
>
> – Des Cummings

The Adventist church's commitment to "the gospel of health" was so deep that they established a health and healing system based in Battle Creek, Michigan, to advance this work. It became the capital of the Adventist health movement. Battle Creek and its citizens benefited by becoming known throughout the nation as "Health City." In 1958 the Loma Linda University School of Public Health, located in California, launched research based on tracking the health habits of Adventist church members. This ongoing longitudinal study continues to advance the science of health and the well-being of all humanity.

Because the Adventist Health System popularized this lifestyle, it is our duty and honor to share it with you. It has been my good fortune to be born into a family that practiced this lifestyle. It is my privilege to offer you a personal tour of these health principles that have become foundational to my life. It is summarized in eight secrets that will give you the best opportunity to experience living as young as possible for as long as possible. My hope is that it will inspire you to imagine living to a Healthy 100.

Many of the health heroes you will meet in this book are part of a group of 90,000 Seventh-day Adventist church members who have been studied for fifty years through grants from many research organizations including the National Institutes of Health (NIH) and the Center for Aging. I refer to this group in two terms—*Adventists* and *All-Stars of Longevity*. While these secrets are derived from the lifestyle of church members, they are based on God's ideal for health that is open to anyone. We invite you to pursue this lifestyle because it is both sensible and scientifically validated. It is not meant to idolize the Adventist church, but it is meant to inspire a nation to envision a healthy future.

The goal of the Adventist Health System is to share these secrets with every community and every patient we serve. Our belief is that these principles provide a healthstyle that, if adopted, could bring the benefits of good health, long life, and reduced health costs to all people. They represent the best personal response that each of us can make to assure our health and the health of our families.

No matter what your faith background or health history, this book was written for you.

Des Cummings Jr., PhD
Executive Vice President
Adventist Health System

1

GO AFTER LIFE

The Spirit of a Healthy 100

I LOVE LIFE!" JOHN'S FACE BEAMS WITH A MILLION-dollar smile as he lifts a bottle of water into the air. "My philosophy for living a full life is to celebrate it every chance I get. So I toast life at every meal. Some people think I'm crazy, but this is the secret that has helped me defy the odds," he says.

"You see, I was born with cystic fibrosis, and when the doctors finally diagnosed it, they told my parents I wouldn't live past age twelve and that my quality of life would be highly compromised," he added. "But here I am at age fifty-three. That's why I celebrate life wherever and whenever I can."

John has the spirit of a Healthy 100. That spirit is the greatest gift I could wish for you. A love for life is what powers the pursuit of a long life. So my first question for you is: *Do you want to live to a healthy 100?*

I believe some of the key factors in John outliving all the predictions of his early demise are his passion for life at home, his love of his work, and his consistent attitude of worship. These have allowed him to surpass the life-limiting conditions that started swirling around him from the moment his mother panicked when he couldn't digest her breast milk. This was just the prelude to a childhood of illness, punctuated by the inability to gain weight and severe recurring stomach cramps.

John's doctors were initially confounded by his condition. So his mother set out on a search for clues to understanding his poor health. One day, as she kissed him on the cheek, she noticed that his skin tasted salty. This clue fit with an article that she had read about cystic fibrosis (CF). The genetic defect that causes CF interferes with the body's ability to move salt in and out of cells, and the salt that cannot be absorbed is excreted through the skin by the sweat glands.

Over the years numerous physicians tried to brace John's family for his early death from this devastating disease that attacks important organ systems, especially the lungs and pancreas. His mother recalls hearing predictions such as:

"He won't live past twelve."

"He'll never be able to attend college."

"He won't have enough stamina to pursue a career."

"He'll likely never live to get married and have a family."

"He won't live past age thirty-five."

But John has surpassed all predictions and all the norms. According to the Cystic Fibrosis Foundation, "In 1955, children with CF were not expected to live long enough to attend grade school." And as recently as 2009 the life expectancy of someone with CF was "in the mid-30s."[2]

Now in his mid-fifties with two children of his own, John Sackett is the CEO of Avista Adventist Hospital in Louisville, Colorado. He lives out his passion for health and healing every day in his life and leadership. He might be the oldest living person with CF, but he doesn't want to know because that fact in itself suggests limitations. Limitations are not his focus.

"I strive to be fully abandoned to joy," John says. This is the spirit of a Healthy 100 person! Life filled with love is worth living. When this reality is yours, you pursue health as the means to extend the joy of living. That's why I want to live to 100!

The question is how? How can I live as long as possible while remaining as young as possible? How can I apply John's secrets to my life? Welcome to the eight secrets of a Healthy 100 and the stories of people who live them! Throughout this book you will be inspired by health heroes who demonstrate how to live "life to the full."

> As I see it, every day you do one of two things:
> build health or produce disease in yourself.
>
> — *Adelle Davis*

You'll meet Rosemary, who lost nearly half her body weight, *one hundred forty pounds* to be exact, and is keeping it off thanks to a changed lifestyle that involves a better diet, more exercise, and an inner commitment to living "life to the full."

You'll meet Brian, whose close encounter with death from heart disease forced a total makeover, including dietary changes, changes in his attitudes, the clarification of his purpose for living, and a commitment to lifelong learning about healthy living in general.

You'll meet Gladys, who at ninety-two became the oldest woman to complete an official marathon.

You'll meet three generations of the Houmann family determined to pass on a legacy of health and generosity to future generations.

Though you may not share the exact same situations, challenges, limitations, abilities, or disabilities as these people, you do share the same opportunity—to live "life to the full." You'll be inspired by their stories and informed by the health principles they practice. And you'll be challenged to implement your own plan for a Healthy 100.

2

Why Would I Want to Live to 100?

Overcoming the Barriers to a Healthy 100

I DON'T *WANT* TO LIVE TO 100!" THE DOCTOR'S strong words caught me off guard. I had asked for an appointment with this highly respected physician to interview him on the secrets of longevity. When I explained that I was writing a book encouraging people to imagine living to a Healthy 100, his response was immediate and charged with emotion. I had to probe deeper. "Why don't you want to live to 100?"

"I don't think I will be able to enjoy life. I'm not looking forward to retirement, much less living to a hundred." My interest was piqued as I noted the rigid body language of fear permeating this middle-aged physician. I leaned forward wanting to hear and understand more.

"Tell me why you are concerned about retirement?" I asked.

He leaned back, folded his hands, and looked at me. I realized this ten-minute interruption between cases was about to expand to a thirty-minute dive into the heart of an overachiever. He started by tackling one of the primary stereotypes of retirement.

"You know, I love golf, and I probably wouldn't mind playing more often. But golf could never replace the fulfillment I find in caring for patients. My greatest moment of personal satisfaction is when I am doing a complicated case that requires all of my focus. My whole being is engaged in the moment as I step through the procedure that could resolve my patient's life-threatening problems. Do you know what it is like to have patients and their families entrust themselves to your care? It is humbling and exhilarating at the same time. But most important, do you know what it is like to make a difference in their health today and provide them with a future of full recovery?" he asked.

> Of all the self-fulfilling prophecies in our culture,
> the assumption that aging means decline
> and poor health is probably the deadliest.
> — Marilyn Ferguson

"All the training and research I have gone through combines with years of experience to prepare me for this moment. I am totally absorbed in the healing process. This is the moment when I feel closest to God and most significant to people. To me, this is worship! And I'm afraid that in a few years I will lose the ability to perform these procedures and will be at risk for losing this deep satisfaction I find in my life and work. In truth, I don't know if I will ever be able to find something as fulfilling as I age, and that is why I don't want to live to 100!"

The nature of the interview had changed. No longer about the science of aging, it was now about the intensity of living "life to the full." We were really talking about the essence of life, and the physician's honesty had surprised us both. I leaned back and took a deep breath.

"So is your greatest fear the loss of significance?" I asked.

"Absolutely," he responded with the decisiveness of a surgeon.

"Are you threatened that you will have to dial down your fulfillment and lose your passion for life?" I inquired.

"No question!"

"Finally, are the options for retirement modeled by your retired colleagues confirming this life sentence of lost significance?" I asked.

"Exactly! I can't imagine a retirement of leisure providing a true sense of purpose. Not in the least!" he replied.

"You have not imagined another passion that could provide you with the same significance that you experience today? And you don't want to simply join the ranks of the good old boys sitting around talking about the good old days?" I followed up.

"Not if I can do better!" he said.

"So if you could find a passion as you age, one that would absorb you and call out the best in your being . . . would you want to live to 100?"At that moment there was a knock on the conference room door. "Come in," the surgeon said.

A nurse popped her head into the room. "Excuse me, doctor. I've been paging you. The team is ready and waiting to start the next case."

"Sorry—got to go. This is a critical case," the doctor said to me. A tone of anticipation filled his voice, and his pace quickened as he left the room. His sense of significance was accentuated by the rehearsal of protocols that began as the nurse accompanied him down the hall. His focused concentration told me he was in the "zone" —the place where everyone is at their best.

As I sat in the conference room, the doctor's objection echoed off the walls, amplified by a cacophony of objections that other people had voiced when I had talked to them about imagining a Healthy 100. I realized that I couldn't ignore those barriers to beginning the journey. So let me add three other objections before I share my conclusions from the doctor's story. Almost all begin with this common phrase: *The Healthy 100 won't work for me because . . .*

- **I've got bad genes!** Do you feel as if you've been dealt a genetic hand that is impossible to overcome? You've already met John, one of my health heroes, who has his sights set on a Healthy 100 despite cystic fibrosis, and whose life models how to exceed genetic limitations.

- **I've got a health-limiting disease!** Perhaps you already have a limiting health condition and are simply hoping to survive this year. You can't imagine an extended life expectancy. If so, you need to read Sheila's story in the chapter about outlook. She was diagnosed with stage four breast cancer at age forty. Learn what question so revolutionized her thinking that her life is now on a completely different trajectory. She set out on an unlikely journey that will inspire you to do the same. Sheila will show you how to borrow hope from others when you are afraid to hope. Every time I read her story I am filled with courage and inspired by her question.

- **I'm too old to start now!** In the chapter on Activity you'll learn about Gladys who completed a marathon at age ninety-two. Gladys's gift for inspiring others doesn't stop with exercise and adventure. She also gives of herself to help those in need and encourages others to do the same. In her story you'll learn about her secret motivation and the unexpected results she achieved.

THE CORE QUESTION

Let's go back to my encounter with the physician. As I watched the doctor disappear down the hall I realized he had articulated the core question that must be answered to achieve a Healthy 100 lifestyle:

"Why do you want to live to a Healthy 100?"

The distress he fears most is one all of us should share—the diminishment of meaning. I have concluded that the most threatening aspect of aging is not slowing down, but numbing down. It's losing your sense of contributing to (or providing) something significant that will change the world. It's experiencing a diminishing zest for life when you stop doing work that is deeply meaningful.

To address this fear and inspire you to imagine a Healthy 100, I realize that this book must go far beyond diet, weight management, and exercise. It must provide you with a lifestyle model that will engage your body, mind, and spirit. It must address both science and significance.

It must answer the doctor's question: *Why would I want to live to 100?*

It must be able to provide you with a model of both why and how to live to 100. It's my desire to introduce you to "Passionaries" for life whom I have met. They are people who have found their purpose for living. They are filled with a personal sense of mission, a clear vision for how they can make a difference, and a passion to pursue it. That describes Passionaries.[3] Having a sense of purpose that transcends time is the key. My fear is not that you will die before your time but that you will live without meaning. I could not have written this book unless I had found a purpose that transcended time—one that my wife Mary Lou and I could share . . . one that will create a legacy of health and happiness for our children.

I believe that the only legacy greater than the gift of health is the gift of love. "The 8 Secrets of a Healthy 100" will advance your ability to leave both gifts. But the next question is where did these secrets come from? What are they? And why are they more compelling than other secrets of living to 100?

3

WHAT YOU CAN LEARN FROM THE ALL-STARS OF LONGEVITY

Origin of the 8 Secrets

THE TELEPHONE RANG—MY ASSISTANT ANnounced it was Disney Development. I knew that this was the call I had been waiting for. I picked it up and heard, "Congratulations! Florida Hospital has been chosen to be the healthcare provider for the new Disney city of Celebration." The words I had hoped to hear for the past year rang in my ears as excitement engulfed me. A year of creative planning and prayer by an elite team of health leaders was rewarded. Our proposal had been chosen!

The city of Celebration was designed to be the fulfillment of Walt Disney's original dream for EPCOT (the Experimental Prototype Community of Tomorrow). Michael Eisner, the CEO of Disney at the time, had commissioned an extensive planning and research effort that involved world famous architects, community planners, and the renowned Disney Imagineers in designing "America's new home town."

Florida Hospital, along with other nationally leading health organizations, was invited to submit a proposal for creating the "healthiest city in America." Our vision for health was summarized in a sentence, *"Our goal is to create the healthiest city in America, based on the secrets of the healthiest people in America."* The team focused on answering a vital question: *what are the keys to advancing health in the twenty-first century?* Once we were chosen, I felt compelled to ask the Disney team to share the primary reasons for selecting our proposal. They answered by referring me to one of the experts who recommended our proposal—Dr. Ken Pelletier. At the time Dr. Pelletier was Stanford University's renowned health and wellness expert. As I listened to his insights, I concluded that Dr. Pelletier recommended our proposal because:

1. Adventists wrote the book on modern health and wellness. Their health system was founded in 1866 with a mission to improve the health of America.

2. The National Institutes of Health (NIH) funded research. In 1958 the NIH began to fund research focused on the Adventist lifestyle. The research demonstrated that this lifestyle produces a longer and healthier life.

3. This study has been replicated with Adventist populations around the world, producing similar health benefits.

For these reasons and more Dr. Pelletier supported the recommendation that Florida Hospital be chosen as the best partner to help the citizens of Celebration achieve their health potential.

Why is the longitudinal study referenced above so significant? The Adventist Health Study has been in existence for over fifty years and has continued to add new subjects. The findings have demonstrated that the benefits of this lifestyle are not limited to a specific religious or ethnic group but can apply across race, gender, and culture. Given these factors, I believe that as you examine the

8 Secrets of a Healthy 100 you will find they can help you reach your health potential as well.

HOW WILL WE MAKE HISTORY?

After being chosen, our next step was to begin the work of designing the "healthiest city in the world." The Disney Imagineers are known for doing things that are magical and world changing. They challenged us to do the same as we planned a hospital that would be able to provide excellence in both health and healing. Our creativity soared as we focused on answering a vital question: *What are the keys to advancing health in the twenty-first century?* We concluded that the most compelling answer would be found by combining the best of the past with the opportunities of the future.

> If you ask what is the single most important key to longevity, I would have to say it is avoiding worry, stress and tension. And if you didn't ask me, I'd still have to say it.
>
> – George Burns, who lived to 100

To define the opportunities of the future we invited a group of health futurists and luminaries from around the world to join our team for a three-day planning symposium on the future of health. A task this momentous had to be convened at the Magic Kingdom—it was a setting that stimulated ideas. The timing was right, in that Celebration was scheduled to open just four years before the dawn of the twenty-first century. As the thought leaders from various countries shared their hopes that Celebration would become a model for health, they also expressed great concern that the combination of unhealthy lifestyles, chronic diseases, and aging would converge to plunge the world into a health crisis. New ways of improving healing and inspiring health were required. We had the opportunity to create a model for the world. The symposium was challenged by the hope of health and the fear of an impending crisis of disease. These dual forces created an urgency that produced three intense days of visioning. The mind-bending solutions for creating the hospital of the future were recorded in story form and illustrated by a graphic artist on 4'x 8' paper billboards and summarized in a thirty-page booklet that launched our journey to make history.

THE BEST OF THE PAST

To mine the rich legacy of health from our past, we returned to the founding documents of the Adventist Health philosophy—an exhilarating journey. I think you will find the highlights fascinating.

In 1866 in Battle Creek, Michigan, the Adventist Health System was chartered with these words, "The proper way to avoid disease, or to recover from it, is to adopt correct habits of life. We pledge ourselves to live in accordance with these principles and will use our best endeavors to impress their importance on others."[4]

This call for lifestyle medicine founded on scientific principles was advocated by health visionaries Ellen and James White. James's passion for this mission was based on personal experience. A series of mini-strokes disabled White in his mid-thirties, and he was forced to take a leave of absence from his role as president of the Seventh-day Adventist church. His wife took him to the doctors of the day, and they offered bleeding, leeching, and drugging as the healing solution. She refused these treatments in favor of following her vision of health founded on natural remedies such as exercise, fresh air, sunshine, water, and a vegetarian diet. Through his wife's nursing efforts, augmented by physicians who practiced these principles, James White was able to regain his health in the span of eighteen months.

Instead of returning to his role as president of the church, James White focused on launching a health ministry. He encouraged the young church to embrace health as one of the core benefits of the Christian life. The Whites embraced the cause of health with the conviction that America desperately needed health reform based on God's plan for natural living integrated with the science of modern medicine. Therefore the first medical facility based on this philosophy was named the Western Health Reform Institute. Opening in June 1866, the health and

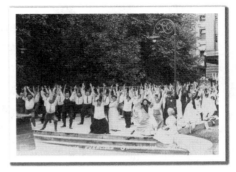

Exercise and Breathing Class outside the Battle Creek Sanitarium [Photo Courtesy of Willard Library — Battle Creek, Michigan]

healing ideas experienced rapid adoption, and later the institution became known as the Battle Creek Sanitarium and Hospital.

To ensure that the movement would be founded on solid medical science, the Whites encouraged many young people to enter the medical profession. They personally sponsored John Harvey Kellogg, a promising young man who would become the leading physician of this health reform movement. John fully embraced Ellen White's vision of health and set out to advance it. The impact of his health and wellness leadership was featured in a recent edition of the *Journal of the American Medical Association*:

> *Kellogg was without question one of the most famous physicians in the United States . . . During his storied career, hundreds of thousands of persons with serious illnesses ranging from cancer and cardiac disease to gastric ulcers and debilitating digestive disorders demanded Kellogg's treatments, which combined modern medicine, surgery, and bacteriology with an eclectic blend of hydropathy, vegetarianism, exercise, and spiritual*

uplift." Those seeking treatment included "such luminaries as John D. Rockefeller Jr. . . . Thomas Edison and Henry Ford, whenever they were in need of a tune-up or recharge from the stresses of industrial gigantism; Amelia Earhart, before her important flights; Warren G. Harding, before embarking on his presidential run; and Booker T. Washington and Sojourner Truth, nursing wounds fresh from fighting the war against racism . . . A vegetarian long before the term was coined, Kellogg developed his dietetic theories in protest against that era's standard fare of fatty, salted meats and fried foods. One of Kellogg's most popular books, Tobaccoism, was published in 1922 and is considered by many medical historians to be the first popular text alerting Americans to the dangers of tobacco smoking . . . In his day Kellogg was the industrial king of wellness.[5]

Physicians and nurses trained at Battle Creek launched a health movement that birthed many of today's five hundred Adventist hospitals and clinics around the world. The movement had such an impact that Battle Creek became known as "Health City."

Health City! That's exactly what we wanted for Celebration . . . to have it recognized as a health mecca, attracting people from around the world. Our team set out to understand the keys to developing a city with a health culture.

We found that many of the health benefits we enjoy today can be traced to this health reform movement. For example, Dr. Kellogg viewed proper nutrition as a key to health and set out to improve America's food choices. Many of his patients were suffering from life-threatening digestive and cardiac diseases, and he traced the problem to unhealthy high-fat American breakfasts. His first nutritional solution was granola. Manufactured in the sanitarium's experimental kitchens, it became quite popular. But it was Dr. Kellogg's invention of corn flakes that truly birthed the cereal industry. Doctor Kellogg's brother W.K. (Will Keith) Kellogg had the vision and business acumen to popularize the Kellogg's cereal brand around the world, and it remains a global leader today. If you are like me, you're benefiting from this breakfast reform break.

The health breakthroughs didn't stop with cereal but spread (pardon the pun) to peanut butter, soy milk, and meat substitutes. They went beyond nutrition to exercise equipment, including the rowing machine, stationary bicycle, weight machines, the mechanical horse, and the dynamometer—a machine designed to measure muscle strength that proved so valuable it was adopted by the military. The program advanced to include aerobics and became, in conjunction with Columbia Records, the first to set exercise to music; the regime also included proper breathing and posture instruction. Battle Creek offered a variety of spa services, including massage therapy, weight loss, and over two hundred forms of baths.

THE 8 SECRETS

Armed with the history of Health City, we were ready to begin planning health into Celebration and designing the hospital of the future. Celebration's lead architect, Robert A.M. Stern, dean of the Yale School of Architecture, challenged us to capture the Battle Creek secrets of healthy living in a few key concepts that could be *archithemed* into the building. He explained that the most powerful buildings are those shaped by a theme that captures the core philosophy behind the mission of the organization. The Florida Hospital team began the process of summarizing the rich history and health principles of our past.

It soon became apparent that the essential concepts of our pioneers could be traced to one source—the biblical story of creation. Over and over these health reformers grounded their advice in the pattern of living that was portrayed in the Garden of Eden—from a vegetarian diet, pure water, physical activity, fresh air, smoke- and drug-free living, to one day a week set aside for time with God and family. They were convicted that this Eden story contained the original model of health, and they set out to translate it into a lifestyle. Another creation perspective that was foundational to the pioneers' philosophy was the conviction that true health was dependent on vitality of the body, mind, and spirit. The mind and spirit have profound influence for advancing health or disease. Therefore, it is critical to embrace a whole-person view of health.

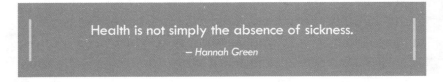

Health is not simply the absence of sickness.

— *Hannah Green*

Finally, our health design team devoted hours of research to summarizing the principles of health in the creation story. The result was eight principles of health from the seven days of creation that summarized the major elements of Adventist health philosophy. These eight principles are expressed in an acronym that spells the word CREATION. They form the eight secrets of a Healthy 100.

C – **Choice:** The first step toward improved health is making consistent healthy choices, which turn into habits and ultimately lead to lifestyle improvement.

R – **Rest:** More than getting a good night's sleep, healing rest means making space in your day to relax and taking a day once a week for restoration.

E – **Environment:** We were made for a garden, but we live in a jungle. Environment is the space outside of us that affects what happens inside of us.

A – **Activity:** There are three kinds of physical activity and three dimensions to physical activity. Combine them, and you're on your way to optimum health.

T — **Trust:** Our faith, beliefs, and hopes affect our health. A trusting relationship with the Creator empowers and enriches every aspect of life.

I — **Interpersonal:** Positive relationships contribute to good health, while toxic relationships can destroy it. So seek to give and receive unconditional love.

O — **Outlook:** Outlook not only colors your perspective on life, but research suggests attitude can influence your health and even impact the progression of disease.

N — **Nutrition:** Food is the fuel that drives your whole system. Eat for energy, eat for mental clarity, eat for longevity. After all, your health is worth it.

ARE THE 8 SECRETS MY BEST HOPE FOR A HEALTHY FUTURE?

In 2005 longevity research specialist Dan Buettner was commissioned by *National Geographic* to identify and study the healthiest people in the world and produce a special edition entitled "The Secrets of Longevity." Buettner concluded that there were several populations around the world with the longest life expectancy. The winners were: the Sardinians in Italy, the Okinawans in Japan, and the Seventh–day Adventists in Loma Linda. He dubbed the Adventists America's "Longevity All-Stars" because they live longer than the average American (on average eleven years) and produce more people who live to one hundred than any other American lifestyle. That's good news! Because by applying these eight health secrets to your life, you too can become a Longevity All-Star. But that is not the end. I believe there is much more opportunity than to advance life expectancy from seventy-eight to eighty-nine years. That is the achievement of the all-stars of the past. I believe that these eight secrets provide a compass for charting a lifestyle for breaking the age barrier—the magic number is one hundred. I invite you to join me in advancing the frontier of healthy living to one hundred. We can go beyond "All-Stars" and become "Champions of Health." Together we can launch a movement that will lead health reform in the twenty-first century!

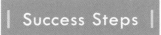

| **Success Steps** |

- **Compare Yourself to the All-Stars of Longevity** – Visit the web site: Healthy100.org and complete the longevity calculator. This will give you a starting point to better understand your health future should you continue with your current lifestyle.

- **Analysis** – Do a "gap analysis" on the results between your longevity score versus the Longevity All-Stars score. That is, notice the gap—if one exists—between where you are and where you want to be. Become a Healthy100 member and receive added support to advance your health.

- **Learn** – Study the eight principles for healthy living as practiced by the Longevity All-Stars. These principles are easily remembered as the CREATION Health acronym. You can learn these principles from reading this book or by going to the web site CreationHealth.com where you'll also find information about our Creation Health seminars.

- **Plan** – Create your own plan based on the CREATION Health principles. Your plan will include areas in which you can make more positive lifestyle choices to change your health future. With this new plan you'll be on your way to imagining a Healthy 100.

4

CHOICE

*First We Make Choices,
Then Choices Make Us*

"DESTINATION, PLEASE," THE VOICE FROM THE GPS requested as I sorted through my folder of papers looking for the location of the conference I was scheduled to address. Seconds later the voice repeated, "Destination, please." This time the GPS added instructions on how to enter information. After several attempts, I finally found the address, entered the destination, and exited the rental car lot. Then a stream of navigation prompts began as my cell phone rang with a call from the office. Now I had two voices to attend to and, as a result, I missed my exit. Frustrated by the fear of getting lost, I hung up the cell phone and heard the GPS voice comment, "Recalculating route." Moments later the navigator's instructions got me back on course.

Life has something in common with a GPS device. To gain optimum value you need to have chosen a destination. This is the first and most significant choice you make. If I were sitting across from you right now, I would ask you to talk to me about your destination, your purpose, or your calling. For Patrick Henry it was liberty; for Martin Luther King Jr. it was freedom and equality; for Mother Teresa it was healing lepers; for Linda Starnes it is helping disabled children; and for Penny Jones it is loving children who need the safety of a foster parent. Have you found your own purpose or calling?

Aristotle suggests a place to look: "Where your talents and the needs of the world cross is your calling." Are you at the point of transition where life has changed and the destination needs to be reset?

THE POWER OF CHOICE

"Have you heard about Rosemary?" It seemed like everywhere I went people wanted to tell me the story of this healthcare case manager who was in the midst of an amazing health makeover. From Dave, my trainer, to Doug, her coach—the buzz was pervasive and the message simple, "You've got to meet Rosemary." So I scheduled a time to listen to her story, and I knew immediately that I had to share it with you in her own words:

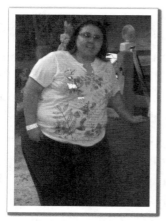

Rosemary before her Healthy 100 lifestyle change

I can't remember a time when I wasn't overweight. In fourth grade I was required to have a school physical, and after they put me on the scale, I was classified as heavy. That was what I expected, because I come from a family of overweight people. Over time as I continued to put on weight I resigned myself to the idea that I was a victim of the "fat gene," and obesity was my destiny. That self-fulfilling prophecy came true, and I continued to put on pounds until I tipped the scale at two hundred eighty-five—that's fifty-

seven pounds for every foot of height (I'm five feet tall).

As a healthcare worker I was aware of the risks of obesity, but simply put, I didn't find anything that would slow my steady march to a future of poor health. I had tried to exercise and diet but all to no avail. However, a visit to my relatives in Colombia brought me to a moment of truth. First, I saw a different health pattern—most of them were not obese and some were models of fitness. Second, they confronted me with the fact that I needed to do something to lose weight.

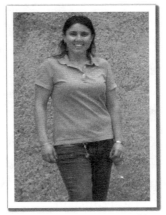

Rosemary after her Healthy 100 lifestyle change

Over my stay, different family members talked to me about how heavy I was getting and encouraged me to lose weight.

When I returned home I went to the doctor and asked if I was a candidate for bariatric surgery. Over the next few months the insurance company approved my request for surgery. I was certain that this was the only way to deal with my genetic predisposition. In order to prepare for surgery I had to lose twenty pounds, and that is what caused me to become a member of the Celebration Health Fitness Center.

Doug Parra, the exercise physiologist and former professional soccer player who teaches Mind, Body Wellness Camp, encouraged me to try his program, and to my surprise I began to lose weight. Over the first month I lost twenty pounds, and Doug encouraged me to push my surgery back for one month and see if the weight loss would continue. I did, and the pounds continued to melt away. The key was a "choice" makeover. My self-talk changed, and I began to imagine that I could achieve a healthy weight. My spirit was filled with hope. My friends were a key as they joined me in the classes and encouraged me every day. My food choices changed, and it transformed my kitchen cupboards. My exercise pattern moved from a dreaded obligation to a healthy habit I enjoyed. And people began *to notice—I was free from my imagined genetic limitations of a life of obesity. I was free from the idea that surgery was my only hope.*

I have become a model of CREATION Health, and it has changed my life. Twelve months after I began this journey I weighed 145. I had lost almost half my weight. Today I still weigh 145. Choice is the freeing power that has changed me, and I know it can do the same for others. My health goal for the future? I'm imagining a Healthy 100.

One reason Rosemary's story is so powerful is that it demonstrates how she gained control over her situation by exercising her power of choice. At first Rosemary lived in a cycle of frustration. She couldn't imagine losing weight, so she had no motivation to focus on food choices and exercise. Once she practiced what was unnatural for her at the time, new habits developed, and she could envision her goal. When she was finally able to imagine her goal, it motivated her to continue making healthy choices day-by-day. She felt in charge of her health and became a victor instead of a victim.

The power of choice, driven by a compelling goal, is the essence of what moves us toward healthy habits. That power is so significant that it would be irrelevant to tell you about these health habits if you were controlled by instinct and didn't have the freedom to make your own choices.

CHOICE AND YOUR HEALTH DESTINY

It's vital that you understand how much your daily choices influence your health destiny. While genes have influence that is profound for some people, in general your power of choice is three times as powerful as the influence of your genes.[6] Perhaps life has dealt you some bad genetic cards, but those cards do not make up your whole hand. Imagine that you are playing a game that involves a hand made up of twelve cards. You are required to keep three cards—no trade-ins, no discards—but you are free to choose what you want to do with the other nine. That would give you a lot of freedom to determine how to put together a winning hand. Your health destiny works in a similar way. The more your genes have limited your health, the more important it is to make the best health choices possible.

> Remembering that I'll be dead soon is the most important tool I've ever encountered to help me make the big choices in life. Because almost everything...fall(s) away in the face of death, leaving only what is truly important.
>
> — *Steve Jobs*

A fulcrum is the point where a seesaw balances. Move the fulcrum, and a little weight on one end can move a big weight on the other. It's a question of leverage. Archimedes said, "Give me a lever long enough and a fulcrum on which to place it, and I will move the world." Choice is the fulcrum with which you can leverage optimum health. Day-by-day and choice-by-choice you write your own health destiny. The first principle of living to a Healthy 100 is making healthy choices. It is founded upon the first freedom that God gave to humans—the freedom of choice. True love requires freedom of choice. This is why God made choice the centerpiece of the Garden of Eden. The creation story highlights the importance of choice with these words, "In the middle of the garden were the tree of life and the tree of the knowledge of good and evil" (Genesis 2:9). From the beginning, choice has been a key component of life. Choice is not only the first of the eight secrets of CREATION Health, it is the key to practicing the remaining seven.

THE MYTH OF HELPLESSNESS

Too many people believe the myth that their health is genetically predetermined and there's not much they can do about it. It's kind of learned helplessness. However, research into the science of aging is debunking this myth. Dr. Kenneth Cooper of the Cooper Clinic points out, "Longevity is based on about three-quarters lifestyle and one-quarter genes. If you can control the way you live, you can control the way you age."

The landmark ten-year study by the MacArthur Foundation shattered the stereotypes of aging. We now know that 70 percent of physical aging, and about 50 percent of mental aging, is determined by lifestyle . . . the choices we make every day. Rather than being a process of steady decline, aging can be a time of growth—physically, intellectually, socially, and spiritually. The recent research on aging indicates that it's possible to live long without significant disability if we maintain our physical and mental skills, reduce our risk for disease and injury, and stay productive and engaged in life.[7]

> The strongest principle of growth lies in human choice.
> – *George Eliot*

Healthiness is all about habits. Aristotle taught, "We are what we repeatedly do. Excellence, then, is not an act but a habit." Habits can either enslave us or free us. Nathanael Emmons, a prominent seventeenth century American who lived to age ninety-five said, "Habit is either the best of servants or the worst of masters. Bad health habits encumber us, enslave us, and ensnare us, preventing us from moving forward in our lives. On the other hand, good habits are our best friends. We perform them unconsciously, so they move us in the right direction on auto-pilot, and we're free to concentrate on other useful endeavors." [8]

So how can you and I transform poor health habits into good ones? Before we explore the process I would like to ask you to select a poor habit that you would like to transform. Got it? Write it in the blank: _____ .

OK, now let's transform.

HOW TO CHANGE A BAD HABIT

A habit is a recurrent, often subconscious or automatic pattern of behavior that is acquired through frequent repetition. So how can you change something that you have been doing over and over again for a long period of time? Over the past thirty-five years I have worked with people to help them develop healthy habits for life. As a result, I have discovered a transformation process that has helped me and many others answer this question. This is not a Cinderella strategy that works instant change; instead, it's a butterfly strategy that wraps you with an environment in which the "caterpillar habit" that holds you down morphs into a "butterfly habit" that lifts you up.

FIVE STEPS TO CHANGE A HABIT

1. The Law of Becoming

The Law of Becoming describes the sequence of developing a habit. In Scripture, the apostle James reveals the anatomy of a habit. He asserts that a habit is conceived in desire, grows in imagination, is born in action, and matures in repetition (see James 1:14–15). The Chinese expressed this law in a proverb: *Sow a thought, reap an action. Sow an action, reap a habit. Sow a habit, reap a destiny.* We have all experienced this pattern. For me it works like this:

I walk through a shopping mall and suddenly the sweet smell of cinnamon pastries stimulates my desire. I am drawn by this powerful scent magnet to gaze at a display of freshly baked cinnamon rolls. My mind begins a bargaining process trying to rationalize the consumption of this treat. *Maybe I can go to the gym tonight and work off the extra calories, I tell myself.* But I know better, so I try to resist. I attempt to walk by the display as though I am not interested. Yet even though my feet are moving, they are slowing down, and I feel the pull of that wonderful aroma. Somewhat conflicted, I step up to the counter and order—perhaps even muttering a self-justifying comment such as, "I hardly ever treat myself. I deserve this!" As I sit down and take a bite I let the mixture of cinnamon spice, freshly baked roll, and creamy frosting dance across my taste buds. (Now you know my weakness and how I fall off the health wagon.) Did you notice the progression I went through? Let's take a closer look.

The key to understanding my cinnamon roll habit is that it engaged my whole person. It began with the body as the smell surrounded me. It advanced to the mind as I rationalized this exception. It culminated in the spirit as I imagined the experience. Finally, I took the step of indulging in something I knew I shouldn't.

But wait . . . once you understand how this process works, it can be used to develop good habits as well. It's important to know, however, that you can't create a habit that sticks by simply applying a "body" strategy. This is why diets are so ineffective for most people. They try to force the body to do something that the mind and spirit aren't in sync with.

Rosemary realized that fact and decided on a lifestyle change, not just a diet. Her wake-up call came when her doctor told her that based on her current condition she wouldn't live past sixty. You can't start with what you need to do unless you have determined why you need to do it. Rosemary's why was to live a long and healthy life. She set out to find out how she could do that and chose the eight secrets of a Healthy 100.

2. The Practice of Substitution

The way Rosemary overcame each of her bad health habits was to substitute a good health habit in its place. What new habit would you like to develop in place of your current unhealthy habit? To be successful, your new habit must be something that you want more than the old habit. Most people fail to implement this powerful law. Instead they adopt the practice of subtraction versus substitution. They focus on stopping an old habit instead of starting a new one. Then they wonder why they always return to the old behavior. Dr. Luke records the frustration of this strategy in Luke 11:24–26. He describes how the subtraction approach can leave you worse off than before you started. It is this mistake that sets many people up for failure.

> Habit is either the best of servants or the worst of masters.
> — *Nathanael Emmons*

Habit reversal therapy, developed by Azrin and Nunn in 1977, illustrates the power of substitution. A nurse research team applied this practice to patients who were suffering from skin conditions that caused them to itch. When the patients scratched themselves, they further aggravated and advanced the disease, leading to a habitual cycle of itching and scratching. Patients had to change the harmful scratching response in order to be healed. The team tried to practice subtraction by admonishing patients to stop scratching every time they noticed this behavior. This strategy was a total failure, frustrating both the nurses and the patients. But when they applied the practice of substitution by helping patients to focus on a more healing behavior, they were able to achieve remarkable results. [9]

Here's the point: you can't achieve positive change with negative goals. So for most people it doesn't work long-term to say, "I won't eat *this*" or, "I need to stop doing *that*." It creates a habit hole that is aching to be filled. Instead, try substitution. By identifying and prizing a positive goal, you not only provide powerful motivation for yourself but also a method for change.

If you visit the web address Healthy100.org/Anger you will find a helpful case study focused on transforming anger along with a healthy habits worksheet. These tools will help you apply this strategy for transforming your habits. The key is to engage your mind, body, and spirit because habits affect the whole person—so the substitution practices must also encompass the whole person.

I've found that habit change strategies are most effective when they are holistic. Remember Rosemary's victory? In her mind she substituted, "I have the fat gene—and I can't change" with, "Healthy choices can make a difference—I'm not predestined to be fat." In her spirit she moved from "anger, guilt, and discouragement" to "hope and prayer for power to keep going." She told me she prayed with every push-up, and she sought the support of healthy friends. In her body she substituted unhealthy foods and little exercise with healthy foods and daily exercise. This approach changed her life, and it can change yours. You can say no to that old unhealthy habit because you have said yes to a new health-enhancing habit, and now you have activated the power of a positive yes.[10]

3. The Practice of Repetition

Have you heard the expression "practice makes perfect"? This was my mother's admonition when she was encouraging me to learn piano. It was also the golf pro's advice when I took lessons to improve my game. However, my golf instructor had a slight variation that pointed out the importance of choosing the right methods. He added one word to my mother's admonition, "Perfect practice makes perfect." His focus was on choosing the right methods and then practicing them. Practicing poor methods yields few good results and great frustration.

The same is true in health. This book is based on eight practices of people who live longer and better lives. Adopting these practices will enable you to transform your poor habits into good ones.

Any new behavior seems very foreign when we first try it. This is because all change processes are foreign to our patterns of feeling, thinking, and acting. It is only through intentional repetition that these actions become ingrained in our mind, natural for our bodies, and congruent with our emotions. Some have tried to document the number of repetitions that are required to create a new habit. Dr. Maxwell Maltz developed the popular twenty-one-day theory of habit formation, and others have proposed numerous other formulas. But scientific studies are inconclusive on how long it will take you to develop these habits. One thing is clear, however—the development of new habits requires repetition.

In a *New York Times* article Janet Rae-Dupree notes, "Brain researchers have discovered that when we consciously develop new habits, we create parallel synaptic paths, and even entirely new brain cells, that can jump our trains of thought onto new, innovative tracks . . . . But don't bother trying to kill off old habits; once those ruts of procedure are worn into the hippocampus, they're there to stay. Instead, the new habits we deliberately ingrain into ourselves create parallel pathways that can bypass those old roads."[11]

In light of this research, the most appropriate advice is to practice until you create a new Healthy 100 bypass in your brain. In short, our goal is to help you build new highways of health, starting in your mind. Our method is based on the apostle Paul's advice, "Do not be overcome by bad, but overcome bad with good."[12]

4. The Practice of Affirmation

An important component of Rosemary's success was the social support she received. In fact, it was critical. Many people who have successfully changed health habits find this to be true. Having a network of relationships with cheerleaders and encouragers along the journey of developing new habits provides great value. From trainers to coworkers you can surround yourself with a circle of friends who offer affirmation. Research chronicled in the book *Vital Friends* found that if your best friend eats healthy you are five times more likely to eat healthy.[13] In a later chapter of this book we will explore the importance of interpersonal relationships, and we will expand on the relationship between your friends and your health.

A second dimension of affirmation is to set times to celebrate the progress of your journey to health. Don't wait to celebrate until you have achieved your big goals. Celebrate small wins! Make every step of your journey to a healthy 100 an opportunity to express joy and gratitude.

> A man too busy to take care of his health is like a mechanic too busy to take care of his tools.
>
> — *Spanish proverb*

The third and final dimension of affirmation is to tell your story to others. Explain what you have found to be the secrets of change, and inspire others to join you. Sharing will serve as a powerful means of self-affirmation and growth. The education of medical professionals is based on the model of "see one, do one, teach one." Through this method, physicians, nurses, and other clinicians have developed professional habits of practice. By teaching someone else, you will affect yourself, advance your commitment to health, articulate your key learning, and further engrain the new brain patterns that are so critical to bypassing old habits and cementing new ones.

5. The Practice of Recovery

One of the greatest threats to your success is the lack of a recovery plan. God and friends play a vital role here. God provides forgiveness that allows you to put your failure behind you, and friends provide the accountability. They can hold you accountable for continuing to practice your healthy habits, and they can help you get back on track when you slip back into an old rut.

Rosemary told me how she missed some of her training and how critical it was to have Doug call her with encouragement to get back on track. He would also call or text at key times during the day when he knew she was most tempted to get off track. If she had failed he would talk her through the guilt and self-disappointment, enabling her to return to the plan. In the nursing study cited above, the team had to remind patients that 100 percent performance of new "non-scratch" behaviors was not the measure of success. They defined success as increasing the practice of healthy behaviors while recognizing that relapses may occur.

In my work helping people to practice recovery I have created a paraphrase of a proverb of Solomon to help them remember that success is not measured by the number of times they fall back but by how quickly they get back up and go forward. "The person who is doing things right falls but rises again. The person who is doing it wrong falls down and returns to the old ways."[14] The key is how soon you return to focusing on your goal versus on your mistake. Falling is never final unless you fail to get up! When you fail, don't beat yourself up with guilt. Simply get up with forgiveness. God forgives you, so why not forgive yourself? If God has a plan for dealing with your failure, so should you. You need to talk yourself through how you are going to respond to failure. Remember Winston Churchill's famous axiom, "Success is never final; failure is never fatal; courage is all that counts."

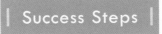

| Success Steps |

• **First Choice** – Why do you want to live to a Healthy 100? What is your purpose for living that motivates you to be your best every day? Write out you personal mission. If you need help go to Healthy100.org/MyMission.

• **Vital Choices** – What are the three most significant choices you need to make to improve your life? Rosemary made some hard choices. List up to three choices she made, based on her story, and then consider (and write down) how you might make these same choices if you had to do so.

• **Five Steps to Change a Habit** – If you struggle with your weight and all the choices that are related to that, what might you do to make better choices more easily and consistently, long-term?

• **Change** – List helpful ideas or guiding principles related to choice and change that you have learned in this chapter. Choose one principle that you will implement as soon as possible in your effort to experience better health.

• **Plan** – Your desire to choose better health will be more successful if you have a plan and especially if you have a plan that takes things step by step. So what is you first step going to be? And your second . . . and maybe even your third? Write these down, and also write down when you plan to take the first step.

• **Obstacles** – Of the five steps to change a habit, which has been the most difficult for you to put into practice? What can you do to overcome that obstacle to your better health?

• **Teach** – If you wish to share your story with others, start a journal, keeping track of all successes and celebrations of each one, with a goal of helping someone else with a similar challenge someday.

5

REST

*We Live with Stress,
But We Don't Have to Die From It*

DOCTOR, THE HELICOPTER IS LANDING. WE'RE ready to transport Mrs. Young."

"But I'm not having a heart attack," Vanessa protested. "I can't be having a heart attack. There's no history of heart disease in my family."

The doctor's calm response downplayed the anxiety that stalked his mind, "We're just going to fly you down to the main hospital and run some tests to make sure." Faith Flight One—Florida Hospital's emergency cardiac transport helicopter—rose from the pad for the ten-minute flight for life. Vanessa had no idea of the gravity of her situation.

She was a high-energy executive for a national public relations firm with responsibilities for sales in the southeastern US. She didn't have time for this unnecessary diversion from critical work. She considered herself to be health gifted—right genes, right health habits, okay (mostly) health habits. She had grown up practicing the health habits of the All-Stars of Longevity:

Nutrition – she was a vegetarian for the most part

Activity – as much as a traveling professional can work into a busy schedule

Environment – she had lived a smoke-free, drug-free life.

Her family had a history of living into their nineties, and she intended to do the same. "I can't be having a heart attack," she stated emphatically, trying to make her point to the medical flight team even as the helicopter lifted off the pad.

The denial process continued until the tests revealed that "Van," as her friends called her, had experienced a heart attack. Her physicians identified at least one significant culprit—not genes, not diet, not lack of exercise or smoking, but STRESS!

REST-ORATION

Van's return to heart health would require replacing unhealthy stress with healthy rest of the spirit, mind, and body. In a word, she needed restoration.

Her plan began by renewing her commitment to experience a weekly day of rest—the kind that is described in the seventh day of creation. This is a strategy that world-renowned longevity researcher, Dan Buettner, identified as the number one health secret you can learn from the All-Stars of Longevity. In his bestselling book The Blue Zones, he gives the following advice:

> *Create a sanctuary in time, a weekly break from the rigors of daily life, the 24-hour Sabbath provides a time to focus on family, God, camaraderie, and nature. Adventists claim this relieves their stress, strengthens social networks, and provides consistent exercise."*[15]

If there was only one health habit that I could emphasize, it would be to create your own sanctuary in time, a weekly vacation from life's daily stresses—a time to relax and grow in love with your family.

MODERN LIVING REQUIRES A "SANCTUARY IN TIME"

Stress is a normal part of everyday living. Throughout our lives, all of us have varying degrees of stress. Stress can affect every part of us. There are healthy and unhealthy ways to deal with stress. Healthy ways of dealing with stress help us function efficiently and effectively. They help us think wisely and react quickly when the need arises—at home, at school, on the job, in traffic, and so forth.

Dealing with stress in unhealthy ways can result in non-productive anxiety, and it can lead to chronic stress. It can shorten our lives. Our modern generation is faced with numerous challenges and uncertainties more complex than any other generation. According to a recent survey taken by the Department of Labor, 75 percent of all Americans are constantly plagued by stress. Stress can express itself in the following ways:

> Courage is fear that has said its prayers.
> — *Unknown*

Fear and Worry: Following the September 11, 2001, attacks on the World Trade Center, Jonathan Steinberg, chief of cardiology at New York's St. Luke's–Roosevelt Hospital Center, led a study on New York City's heart patients. He found that they suffered twice the usual rate of life-threatening heart arrhythmias in the months following the attacks. Steinberg observed, "These patients experienced potentially fatal events, even though many of them had trouble identifying themselves as unduly fearful."

Threat Level: In the present day global world, Americans have been at a high threat level for so long that perhaps in order to function, we have repressed our anxiety. But whether it is hidden or not, it affects us! The fact that we are experiencing a concurrent epidemic of stress and cardiovascular disease in America is not a coincidence! Dr. Carol Scott wrote:

> *The heart blood vessels are particularly sensitive to acute and chronic stress. With every beat, the heart not only pumps blood, but transmits complex patterns of neurological, hormonal, pressure and electromagnetic information to the brain and throughout the body. The heart is uniquely positioned as a powerful communication hub that connects the body, mind, emotions, and spirit. There is an elaborate feedback network of hormones, chemicals and nerves that exist between the brain, the heart and centers of thoughts and emotions. The heart sends the brain messages that affect our perceptions, our mental processing and our feelings. It's no surprise, then, that there is a strong connection between stress and cardiovascular health.*[16]

Financial: During the years 2008–2010 the recession had a great impact. According to an Associated Press poll, 46 percent of the people surveyed said they were suffering from debt-related stress. [17]

Sleepless in America: Americans are chronically ill with sleep disorders. Sales of prescription sleep aids have jumped 60 percent since 2000 (with a startling increase among people aged 18–24). The average American is functioning with ninety minutes less sleep than they need for healthy living.[19]

Lack of sleep can do more than make you cranky; it can shorten your lifespan.

Researcher scientists from the UK's University of Warwick recently reported their study of 470,000 people from eight countries and found that the demands of the modern workplace and family are taking a toll. The risk of heart disease can increase as much as 48 percent and the risk of stroke by 15 percent when a person regularly does not get at least six hours of sleep. The researchers found that chronic sleep shortages produce hormones and chemicals in the body that increase the risk of cardiovascular disease.

Always "on" Multitasking: You were not made for a "24/7 always on" multitasking environment. MIT Professor Sherry Turkle studies the impact of technology on our daily lives. "Technology promises to let us do anything from anywhere with anyone. But it also drains us as we try to do everything everywhere. We begin to feel overwhelmed and depleted by the lives technology makes possible."[19]

"We must ruthlessly eliminate hurry from our lives," was the advice that John Ortberg got from a wise friend.[20] Hurry makes you skim life instead of really living it. You never go deep into any experience—a moment of reflection is interrupted by a text message or a schedule alert. Multitasking means you are living several experiences at the same time, under the illusion that more is better as you exchange peace for pace.

You are spurred on by the fear that you may be missing something—the moments of pause when you could relax and refresh are replaced by the compulsive urge to check your messages, text someone, or make a call. The frenetic pace of technology has not released you but enslaved you to living heads-down looking at a screen versus heads-up looking to the sky, the mountains, the soaring of the birds, and the refreshing of your spirit. Even your time of reflection becomes rushed. The problem is that rest is not instant like coffee; it takes time to settle down and live. You wonder why you feel like you have skimmed life—reacting to many things superficially with shorthand living and living few things with all your being. I invite you to assess your rest—Mary Lou and I did just that, and it changed our lives.

YOU WERE DESIGNED FOR SABBATH

Early in our marriage Mary Lou and I studied the health-enhancing power of a weekly Sabbath. Experiencing this twenty-four-hour sanctuary in the week has become a habit that is key to both our health and happiness. It is a physical, mental, and spiritual time dedicated to renewing our love. The idea of taking a day off for love comes from the creation story. On the seventh day God had completed his work, and he simply took the entire day to be with his children. I believe he was telling us that this is the purpose of all of his plan and work. Taking time with God and each other is when we experience the love that is the essence of life.

Love not only enhances health, but many physicians have asserted that it is one of the most powerful forces for healing. In his book *Love and Survival*, Dr. Dean Ornish, a physician known for his work in reversing heart disease, speaks about the power of love. "I am not aware of any other factors in medicine—not diet, not smoking, not exercise, not stress, not genetics, not drugs, not surgery—that has a greater impact on our quality of life, incidence of illness, and premature death from all causes."[21] God intended that our lives would be filled with love, and that is why he gave us a day to experience its benefits.

Based on this belief we have organized our week around a day for love. We dedicate this day to experiencing the three dimensions of love God designed into the perfect day (Genesis 2:2). I guarantee that as you practice these principles love will flourish in your heart.

• **Rest (Trusting Love)**: Rest is a concept rich with meaning. It means to stop and relax in the knowledge that in the end love will win out. This is a huge benefit to your spirit—it provides a sense of security and drives out fear. Mentally, it invites you to set aside the "to do" list and take time "to be." This is God's invitation to simply relax and smell the roses of life. We have found that rest is most important when you hit the rough spots where your week has revealed your weakness. When you have lost a battle and life looks uncertain, you need the realization that God is in control and love will win the war. This realization requires total focus. It is not something that you can multitask. So stop in the name of love! Call a twenty-four-hour time out!

I shared the concept of Sabbath rest in a speech to a group of bankers several years ago. Two years later John, a brilliant lawyer who had attended that meeting, saw me at an event and thanked me for the idea of taking a weekly vacation with God and family. He told me, "It has changed my family life, and we all look forward to spending the day together." It's the perfect plan, and it starts with stopping. Stop the fear, worry, and anxiety of the world

> Step out of the traffic! Take a long loving look at me, your High God, above politics, above everything.
> — Psalm 46:10, The Message

- **Bless (Belonging Love):** To be blessed means realizing God's favor, knowing that God loves you. This knowledge is the root of happiness. In fact the word "blessed" is often translated "happy!" For "the joy of the Lord is our strength." So take a day to experience the happiness that comes from knowing that God loves you and that you love each other. In a world where your self-worth is often under attack, let me summarize the words of Dan Allerton in his book *Sabbath*: " Let the impact of being valued and full of worth drown out the voices of criticism and self-doubt."[22] In our home Sabbaths begin with a special meal, a Sabbath surprise, and a personal blessing. When I bless each person with words of affirmation, it bonds us together in a way that is not achieved by material gifts. Your family is most blessed by the affirmation of your love. It allows them to shed all the pain of loneliness and embrace all of the joy of belonging. Celebrate the blessings of life and the bond of unity with people you love; tell stories; let the joy of life flow throughout your being in laughter.

- **Sanctify (Hoping Love)**: The Hebrew word "sanctify" was used for the engagement of a man and a woman. Engagement is a hopeful ceremony of anticipation, a commitment to a promise of unity and marriage. The third benefit of Sabbath is to bring us into a unity that enables hope in a world where relationships are often shattered and hope is lost. God says, "Come together and repair any cracks in your relationships, reset the fractures in your love for each other. Let my commitment to you bring you forgiving love that will enable you to patch up the breakups in your life." This is God's day to take away the heartbreak in our lives that comes from broken relationships. Failing to deal with the hurts in our lives has severe implications for our health, as Dr. Dick Tibbits documents in chapter six of his book *Forgive to Live*.

Imagine a day each week when you commit to making things right in your family, you take time to celebrate the milestones of love (anniversaries, birthdays, graduations, awards), and you unite to right the wrongs in your world. The result is reconciling love!

SABBATH PRIORITY IN HOLLYWOOD

DeVon Franklin is an executive at Columbia Pictures. His film projects include many successful movies such as the *Karate Kid* remake and *The Pursuit of Happyness*. In his book *Produced by Faith*, Franklin explains the priority he gives to rest: "I celebrate Sabbath. . . . No work. I don't check e-mail or roll calls. I break the fourth commandment of the movie business: *Thou shalt never turn off thy BlackBerry and turn off my BlackBerry.* The Sabbath is my time with the

Lord, my time to unwind from the pressures of work, heal, and reflect on the many blessings in my life. . . ."[23]

While many may find it difficult to discover true inspiration in Hollywood—at least when looking at the real lives of those involved in the film industry—I find DeVon's commitment to Sabbath rest inspiring. Though this young executive was responsible for overseeing film productions with millions of dollars at stake, he chose to set aside twenty-four hours a week to take time to recharge his life and stay connected with God, his family, and his relationships. If a busy Hollywood executive can make Sabbath rest a priority, perhaps it's something any of us could benefit from in our own lives.

PRACTICING REST THROUGHOUT YOUR WEEK

Meaningful work and Sabbath rest are the two secrets to reducing stress in your life, thus advancing health, living longer, and enjoying life more. Life is meant to be lived in a tempo of work and rest.

Return to the tempo of life. To experience it, simply pause to feel the tempo of your being. Place your finger on your pulse, feel the rhythmic beat of your heart. Listen quietly to the tempo of your breathing. Sense your brain waves absorbing the meaning of what you are reading. You were made for a tempo of work/rest. The wave of work/rest is evidence of a healthy heart, brain, and respiratory organs, which can be seen on medical monitors; these are signs of health. A flat line on a monitor is a sign of death.

Does your life flow in a healthy wave pattern, or is it more like a flatline? Flatline living is characterized by pedal to the metal—always on, always busy—multitasking life . . . physically overworked, mentally behind, and emotionally on the edge.

The awareness of the necessity of rest is so pervasive that even some modern machines are being programmed to encourage us to put the rhythm back into our lives. I discovered this for the first time several years ago when I rented a car for an eight-hour road trip. I was focused on making time and planned to stop just for necessities, refueling, restroom, and to pick up food that I could eat while driving. Two hours into the trip this dashboard message appeared, "Rest stop advised every two to three hours." *Interesting but unnecessary*, I thought. An hour later the message reappeared and with flashing insistence. It was a good reminder, one I complied with.

> Unhealthy stress numbs your spirit,
> dumbs your mind, and destroys your body.
> — *Des Cummings*

"Americans . . . we have a pace problem," that car was reminding me. We need more rest stops along the way of our lives. These have been advised by a higher authority than us. The question is whether or not we will pay attention to good advice or have to have a wake-up call like Van had. For many people their first heart attack is also their last heart attack—because they die from it. In Van's case, she had a chance to make some necessary changes.

THE REST OF VAN'S STORY

Throughout her life Van had practiced the principle of Sabbath rest as a wonderful time for family, but following her heart attack it became even more valuable as a time to take a break from the treadmill of stress. Now she embraced it as a day to recover the vital spiritual, mental, and physical benefits of rest that reduce stress. Van recommitted to the 8 Secrets, and she gave special time to service, exercise, and nutrition. The Dean Ornish diet for reversing heart disease became her nutritional Bible.

Recently Van returned to her physician for an annual physical. After all the tests were completed the doctor's verdict was, "You're healthy enough to make it into your nineties."

Van responded, "Doctor, my mother lived to be ninety-six, and I want to at least live to be ninety-five."

The doctor replied, "Really? Well, go for a hundred! You can do it!"

Van decided, "So I'm going to do it. I'm aiming for a Healthy 100! In fact, I'm not only living the 8 Secrets, I am sharing the philosophy with all my friends."

Today Van Young is living "forever young," renewed each week by a day for rest and refreshed each day with rest stops that bring tempo to her living and health to her body, mind, and spirit!

I encourage you to also consider changes to your week. Add a day of rest and restoration. Don't shortchange yourself on sufficient daily rest. Remember that all these choices are yours alone to make. Implement the strategies one-by-one, and watch your level of stress diminish and the rhythms restore your soul.

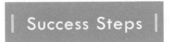

Success Steps

- **You Deserve a Sabbatical** — Plan to experience a weekly Sabbath for you and your family. To assist you in this process go to Healthy100.org/Rest.

- **Overcome the Flatline Schedule** — If you work in an office setting, try working fifty- minute hours. Schedule ten minutes between appointments during which you can summarize the prior meeting, plan follow-up, let your body relax, and clear your mind before the next commitment. This reduces stress by counteracting the nagging thought that you may be forgetting something of importance. If you don't work in an office, consider other ways you can schedule short breaks into your day to clear your mind and release any stress or tension you are experiencing.

- **Improve Your Concentration** – Take an inspiration break—a relaxed moment to listen to music, view nature videos, enjoy a drink (water preferred), have a conversation with God, stretch, or engage in breathing exercises.

- **Get Enough Sleep** – If you're often tired but can't get to sleep (or stay asleep), try changing some of your pre-bedtime routines. Turn off the computer or the TV at least thirty minutes before bedtime. Read a relaxing book for a while after you get into bed. Spend time in Scripture reading, prayer, or meditation with good devotional materials. Keep a worry list and a worry box. Write down those worries, give them to God, then put them in the box overnight. You'll be amazed at how much less worrisome many of these concerns are after a good night's sleep.

- **Refuse to Overcommit** – Read *The Power of a Positive NO*. Align your involvements with your priorities. Block out time for yourself and your family, and make them non-negotiable.

- **Tune in to Your Daily Energy Cycles** – If you hit the wall, say between two and four in the afternoon, take a power nap, or engage in strategic eating by munching some nuts, for example. Skip the caffeine and sugar fixes—they only take you up to let you down.

- **Sanctify Your Day of Rest** – To sanctify something is to set it aside for a specific purpose—in this case to worship, to invest in relationships to renew and restore them, and to advance goodness in your world.

6

ENVIRONMENT

You Were Made for a Garden,
But You Live in a Jungle

BILLY WAS FROM THE ASPHALT JUNGLE OF EAST Los Angeles. His grandparents were attempting to raise him as best they could, but they realized that he needed to get out of that environment if he was going to have a chance to become a productive citizen. So they talked to their pastor who suggested that they send him to Pine Springs Ranch, a summer camp located in the San Jacinto Mountains of Southern California. It would keep him out of trouble and perhaps change his life's direction.

When my phone rang (I was the camp director), the pastor began to explain to me all of the reasons why I should allow Billy to come to camp for eight weeks. I asked him to tell me as much as he knew about Billy's problems at school and in the neighborhood. "I think he is a pretty good kid, but he is headed in the wrong direction," the pastor said. "He is hyper and won't listen to instruction; he gets mad easily, which results in daily fights; he is behind in school and doesn't do his homework. He wanders the streets and comes home at all hours."

"Well, pastor," I replied, "you know we are not a rehabilitation center. You may need to send him to a place that deals with kids who have learning and behavior issues."

The pastor urged me to let Billy come for one week. I agreed to a trial week, and when I hung up the phone I paused to pray for a God-inspired plan to help this troubled child. My mind was drawn to wilderness camp—a special program that taught boys rock climbing, camping, and survival skills. The setting was "skunk cabbage meadows," on the upper slopes of the mountain. Billy would be totally surrounded by a natural environment. At night it was pitch black, and the stars shone with a brilliance undimmed by city lights. The air was high above the smog line, and its crisp freshness made each breath fill your lungs with cleansing purity. The experience made you feel so close to God and so free from stress that the many of the kids who went to "skunk cabbage meadows" didn't want to return to the main camp.

That settled it. I would ask Jack, a college guy whose skills as a naturalist made him a hero to the boys, to take Billy as a personal challenge to see if the God of the mountain could get through to this kid. Jack accepted the challenge with the gung ho spirit of a climber. The trial week was soon extended for the entire summer as the reforming of Billy progressed. Like the metamorphosis of a caterpillar transforming into a butterfly, the cocoon was simply the nature that God had created. Over the course of that summer Billy developed a love for nature and a deep friendship with Jack. The troubled child that came to camp returned reluctantly to the city, but his heart had been captured by the mountain. He had learned the self-discipline of a daily routine where everyone had to do their part, and the teamwork of rock climbing that relied on the support of your partner.

The asphalt jungle was where he lived, but every time he could escape to the mountains he did so. Billy lost his label as a troubled child. What made the difference? Undoubtedly it was his friendship with Jack and the other wilderness campers as well as his newfound relationship with God. But there was one more problem that the camp resolved. It has been called nature deficit disorder.

This label was coined by Richard Louv in his bellwether book *Last Child in the Woods*, the first book to bring together a new and growing body of research indicating that direct exposure to nature is essential for healthy childhood development and for the physical and emotional health of both children and adults. Louv directly links "nature deficient disorder" to some of the most disturbing childhood trends, such as the rise in obesity, attention disorders, and depression. Louv believes that the more we are surrounded by technology, the more we need to be surrounded by nature to keep us mentally, physically, and spiritually healthy. To encourage the connection with nature he has cofounded the Children and Nature Network, which helps families and communities create environments that immerse children in nature.

> Climb the mountains and get their good tidings...
> Nature's peace will flow into you as sunshine flows into trees.
> — *John Muir*

There are a number of studies demonstrating the benefits of children being in nature. One study (American Institutes for Research, 2005) found that students in outdoor science programs improved their science testing scores by 27 percent. Andrea Faber Taylor and Francis Kuo, researchers at the University of Illinois, have shown that the greener a child's everyday environment, the more manageable their symptoms of attention-deficit disorder, and in a report published in August 2008, they described how children concentrate better after a simple walk in the park. Many other studies suggest that children who spend more time in nature are healthier, happier, and better at academic performance.

THE GIFT OF THE GARDEN

God devoted the first four days of creation to fashioning the ideal environment in which humans can thrive—a garden. Fantastic idea! But as the biblical account continues, sin entered and turned our world from a garden to a jungle. So how can we recreate a garden-like sanctuary with the daily demands of our lives?

First of all, we must understand that the greatest effort needs to go into areas of our life that are most jungle-like. Sometimes stress from your day can overload you to the extent that you walk into your home with a predatory mindset as opposed to a peaceful disposition. No matter where you live, try to put aside the jungle atmosphere and create a more garden-like experience. Your home, apartment, or room should be a safe space for you and your family, no predators allowed. If the TV, computer games, DVD movies, office politics, or anything else threaten that peaceful experience, why not remove them from the garden environment you are trying to create?

Here's a rather simple way to recapture the healthy environment of the garden wherever you are. Try taking several "breath breaks" throughout your day.

Proper breathing is the key to delivering life-invigorating oxygen to your vital organs and health-producing energy to your cells. Breath also has a spiritual dimension. The breath of God activated Adam's body, mind, and spirit, and he became a living soul. If you want to live life to the fullest you need to fill your lungs with air as well as refresh your spirit with God's presence. The "breath of God" is synonymous with the Holy Spirit's presence in your life. My breath break improves my health by deep breathing for my lungs and prayer for my spirit. I take this break to refresh my body and restore my soul. I invite you to read the instructions for taking a breath break in the success steps at the end of this chapter.

GARDEN IN YOUR MIND

Our mind is like a garden. We become what we plant and cultivate. I always wondered how Mary Lou was able to hear our children wake up from a nap or cry in the night before I ever heard it. The reason is how she tuned her mind. This is accomplished through our RAS: reticular activating system.

The RAS is a complex collection of neurons, about the size of the tip of your little finger, "that serve(s) as a point of convergence for signals from the external world and from the interior environment."[24] Your brain's unique screening device, it is like a filter between our conscious and subconscious mind. The RAS "is the part of your brain where the world *outside* of you, and your thoughts and feelings from *inside* of you, meet."[25] Here is the beauty—the RAS enables you to plant a sensory garden.

Mary Lou has become my RAS instructor. On our walks or sitting on our porch, she intentionally focuses on the beauty of our surroundings. She speaks of the unique beauty of the cloud formations, the magnolia blossoms, the flowers, the ducks in the lake, etc. She absorbs nature with her whole being by looking at it, touching it, smelling it, hearing it, and speaking it. Then her mind can easily recall it.

When you focus on the beauty around you, your RAS will absorb the image of that environment and plant it in the garden of your mind. In essence we are the keeper of our garden. What we allow to grow in the garden of our mind is our personal choice. God designed the RAS so that we can live in the jungle of this world with the garden on our mind.

MADE FOR A GARDEN

Have you ever wondered why people are drawn to nature's beauty? We don't *do* anything at the Grand Canyon or at the base of a redwood tree; we just take in magnificent natural beauty. Our photo albums include sunsets, mountain peaks, lakes, and beaches. The environment of choice for vacations is most often the lake, the beach, the mountains, or some other wonder of nature.

As I write this I am filled with the anticipation of performing the marriage ceremony of my son Derek and his fiancée, Nalani, on the garden island of Kawai. It's an inspiring spot. Life began in a garden called Eden, which is why I believe that we instinctively know that we were made for a garden, and despite living in a city there is an innate pull of the spirit to get back to the garden where we are free to thrive.

Recreating a healing environment is key to our health, yet it is becoming harder and harder to experience. Part of the reason for this is because, for the past few centuries, humanity has progressively moved away from more rural (nature-filled) environments to cities. This practice has become so prevalent that in 2008, for the first time in human history, more people were living in cities than in rural areas.[26]

While living in cities can certainly have its advantages, there can also be drawbacks. For example, we consider it cruel and unnatural to cage animals, yet we have become accustomed to subjecting humans to the caged world of city life where they often travel underground, surrounded by pollution, consigned to and participating in the "rat race." One of the first impacts of sin was an attack on nature—and this continues today.

Thankfully, many people are taking action to restore nature. For example, some who are committed to the survival of animals have created sanctuaries based in nature preserves where animals can once again thrive. We can do the same for ourselves. We can create nature sanctuaries where garden life is prized and preserved. Whether it is in your home, neighborhood, office, or city—make it your goal to push back the jungle and recreate the garden.

THE JUNGLE EFFECT

The societal change from rural to urban life sometimes brings comments like this one from a friend, "My kids can't relate to a garden as their ideal environment! We never had a garden when they were growing up." In many ways city living has broken the connection between children and nature.

In the open world of my childhood we spent our free time primarily outside, stimulated by the sights and sounds of nature. Sometimes we were disciplined by those awful words, "You have to stay inside." What a change from the way we live now. Today's children are often confined to an inside life stimulated by an electronic environment, living a second life that seems more exciting than their real life. This is unfortunate, because I believe it is critical to the health and well-being of our children that we bring them back to nature. This is why Richard Louv and his colleagues have embarked on a crusade with the battle cry, "No child left inside!"

This principle is not only a key to the health of our children but to the health of adults as well. We were made for a garden, but increasingly people are confined to unnatural workspaces such as cubicles. One-third of workers never go outside during the day. A portion of those who do venture out pollute themselves and the environment by using the escape for a smoking break. Is it any wonder that offices are places of stress, where people get complacent, burned out, and exhausted?

The All-Stars of Longevity are exceptions to this cycle. They may live in the jungle, but they have found ways to recreate garden environments, escapes, and retreats. I invite you to take this path to a Healthy 100 by designing your own personal gardens of health.

HEALTH BENEFITS OF A NATURAL ENVIRONMENT

Today many studies demonstrate how natural surroundings promote wellness, and hospitals and health centers have incorporated nature into interior design and outside areas such as healing gardens. Many other facilities, such as offices and public buildings, also recognize that people are calmer, more focused, and happier in a pleasing natural environment.

> The more high-tech we become, the more nature we need.
> — *Richard Louv*

Designing your environment is called "environmental engineering." It's a relatively new field of study with multiple applications to our topic in this chapter—indeed, to the whole book. The basic idea is that most of us have built into our environment things that tempt us or drag us away from the pursuit of change or the achievement of new goals we might want to achieve in terms of our lifestyle. So for the rest of this chapter I'd like to focus on some environmental engineering ideas for your consideration, each oriented toward avoiding actions that might lead toward failure, while making better choices that will help you successfully pursue health. In all these things, keep in mind that you are not the train; you are the *engineer*. Take positive action. Make changes as you can. Move forward wherever possible. You and your family will be healthier and happier as a result.

Many of the suggestions that follow are drawn from and expanded on in Florida Hospital's book *Creation Health Seminar Personal Study Guide*:[27]

Solar Power

Sunlight is a powerful promoter of health and well-being. Sunlight promotes positive thinking by increasing serotonin, an important "happiness" brain chemical. Reduced serotonin levels have been associated with many disorders including attention deficit hyperactivity disorder (ADHD), irritability, depression, chronic fatigue syndrome, and nausea. Sunlight can kill germs. So just opening your blinds may help you be healthier. While too much sunshine can increase the risk of certain cancers, sunlight in moderate amounts can enhance health. For the best health, it's important to get adequate sunshine without getting sunburned.

Fresh Air

Fresh air is electrified with life-giving oxygen molecules, which enhances a sense of well-being, increases the rate and quality of growth in plants and animals, decreases anxiety through its tranquilizing and relaxing effect, lowers resting heart rate, and decreases survival of bacteria and viruses in the air. Just a partial list of the benefits of cleaning stale air out of our lungs with a breath of fresh air, it may help explain why when you get out into nature one of the first things you do is take a really deep breath! So get outdoors and into nature, especially in areas such as mountains, forests, by the sea, and waterfalls. Also don't forget about the quality of your indoor air. If you live in a place with air pollution, consider an air purifier or add nature's air purifiers, plants, to your environment.

Personal Space

Take a moment to think about your personal space—both at home and in the workplace. Are there windows you can open to let the sun shine in? If not, can you spend at least a little time outside each day? A short walk away from your workspace for some fresh air can be rejuvenating. Can you add some plants or a small table water fountain? Or perhaps you can incorporate beautiful pictures of nature around your home or workspace. These could be photographs for the wall, screensavers on your computer, pieces of art depicting natural scenes and settings, or plasma displays of nature. And what about clutter? Professional organizers advise clients that getting rid of clutter not only makes them more efficient but also creates a freeing sense of energy and mental clarity.[28] Think creatively about a garden environment, and add as many touches of nature as you can.

Aroma

Maybe you've heard the advice that if you're selling your house, you should have the pleasant aroma of cookies or apple pie baking during an open house because it makes potential buyers feel "at home." There may be some truth to this. Our sense of smell can powerfully trigger both positive and negative physical responses. You can use this to your advantage. Is there a particular aroma that brings back a happy childhood memory? Make that a regular part of your environment. Aroma preferences are highly personal (explaining the endless variety of perfumes and colognes), so explore what works for you.

Sound

Does the sound of a dentist's drill set you on edge? What about the sound of ocean waves gently caressing the beach? Sound is an important component of our environment. Research shows that noise elevates psycho-physiological stress (resting blood pressure and overnight epinephrine and norepinephrine), decreases levels of perceived quality of life,[29] and contributes to deficits in long-term memory and standardized reading test scores.[30] Even low levels of noise can reduce productivity.[31] On the other hand, calming music can diffuse the tension caused by noise. Consider including peaceful music into your environment or maybe sounds of nature such as ocean waves or waterfalls on audio.

Getaway

While sound can certainly have a positive influence on our health, the absence of sound can also have a healing effect. Perhaps one of the best escapes we have is solitary quiet. Imagine sitting in the middle of God's garden with only the sounds of nature filling your ears and calming your spirit: birds chirping, a brook flowing gently, the breeze gently rustling leaves. Give yourself time for silence, whether in prayer, meditation, or focusing on a sunrise. I encourage you to turn off the words both outside and inside your head and listen to God's Spirit within. In many ways it seems a conundrum that doing nothing takes practice. But in our fast-paced world it can. See the tools on our website that can help with contemplation that will both relax and energize you. Many studies support the health benefits of meditation. So don't feel like you're doing nothing when you're doing nothing! It's one more piece of a Healthy 100 lifestyle.

START SMALL

Now with all of these ideas, I'm not suggesting you spend a lot of money and overhaul entire living spaces. Just begin with small choices and changes in your effort to move from sensory overload to garden tranquility. Before his death, Henri Matisse, the great modern French painter, spent many months bedridden with colon cancer. His family moved his bed so he could take in the view of the countryside from the window. More importantly, they kept changing what was on his windowsill to continually inspire his creativity. He painted some of his most famous pieces while he was on his deathbed. What a legacy and gift that was to his family and to all who enjoy such genius!

So look around at the spaces you occupy most. Do you find things that inspire you and lift your spirit? Maybe it's just a precious photograph or a simple houseplant. Whatever it is, your surroundings should be about more than just function. Think about sensory experiences that trigger calm and peace for you, and find ways to incorporate them into your environment. You can find more suggestions by visiting Healthy100.org.

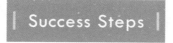

Success Steps

- **Breath Break** — Proper breathing invigorates your body, mind, and spirit. It helps you relax, think more clearly, and have more energy. Take ten minutes a day (or whenever you need a boost) to do the following deep breathing exercise:

  A) Sit or stand comfortably with your back straight, but relaxed; B) Inhale through your nose slowly for a count of four, inflating your belly (not your chest) like a balloon; C) Hold your breath for a count of four; D) Exhale slowly through your mouth for a count of seven, expelling as much air from your lungs as you comfortably can; E) Repeat this exercise three or four times. As your body becomes more used to this activity, you can increase the duration of the breaths or the number of breaths you take. Just be sure to stop if you feel dizzy or faint. To further enhance the experience, use this time of deep breathing to meditate on Scripture or pray silently to God. Once you make deep breathing a regular part of your routine, you may find you get more energy from taking a breath break than from a coffee or snack break.

- **Get Outdoors** — If you work in an office, think of ways you can get outdoors for at least a few minutes every day. Instead of meeting in a conference room with no windows, schedule a walking meeting outside. Read a book outside during your lunch break. Walk around a nearby lake and feed the ducks. Frequent lakeside cafés, have a drink out on the veranda, or enjoy breakfast on the patio.

- **Plan a Special Outing** — Go somewhere or do an activity that will expose you to natural beauty that you've never experienced before. Try camping, canoeing, hiking, climbing, boating, or driving somewhere beautiful. The more you get a picture in your mind of what inspires you in nature, the more you can bring that experience into your everyday life.

- **Get a Pet** — Another great way to experience nature is to get a pet that you can love and nurture. Pet ownership has many documented health benefits. For example, owning a dog may encourage you to take more walks, which has a health benefit on its own. If you live in a place where pets are not allowed, consider getting a membership to a local zoo or volunteering at an animal shelter.

- **Adult/Child Interactions** — Teaching experiences that take place in the environment of nature are often characterized by less stress and more resilience. How about going for an evening walk with your kids and talking through life along the way. Or when discipline is required how about walking and talking through the issue. Perhaps after the discipline you can take a walk together and allow natural healing to take place in the great outdoors as opposed to in the four walls of a room.

- **Indoor Garden** — Many options are available today for creating a small garden within your home. Buy a window box where you can plant seeds to grow a variety of items, including things such as: flowers (marigolds, sunflowers, mums, rainbow mix); vegetables (carrots, celery, onions, tomatoes); herbs (basil, chives, parsley, rosemary). This is also a great activity for kids to be involved in.

HEALTHY 100

7

ACTIVITY

How Activity Fuels Energy and Power-Filled Living

THE EVENT IS THE 2010 HONOLULU MARATHON. The television cameras and reporters are poised at the finish line to capture a long-anticipated world record moment. The exceptional athlete is Gladys Burrill. Trackers have been following her progress throughout the course, and now the finish line spotter identifies her in the distance. The fans lean across the ropes to catch a glimpse of this phenomenon. When she comes into view, cheers break out. Shouts of encouragement fill the air, "Go Glady-ator, go Glady-ator! You can do it! World record! Keep going!"

The previous year she had hoped to set the record only to have those hopes dashed by stomach cramps. But now she is less than three hundred yards from achieving an incredible milestone. Can she keep up the pace? The cheering crowd grows louder.

Suddenly Gladys slows—then stops. The fans' shouts turn to groans, fearing a repeat of last year. Questions fill the air: "Is she injured?" "What's the problem?" "What is she doing?" "Why has she stopped?"

After a minute's pause, Gladys turns the doubts back to cheers as she resumes her pace and crosses the finish line with a world record performance. Her smile tells the story of an incredible journey. Her raised arms evoke cheers from her fans. As she steps forward she is presented with colorful leis and congratulations worthy of a champion.

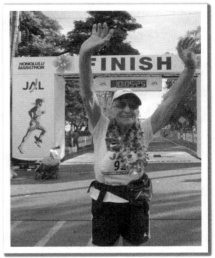

Gladys Burrill completing a marathon at age 92 [Photo courtesy of the Honolulu Marathon]

Gladys Burrill, at age ninety-two, has become the oldest woman to complete an official marathon, with a fast walking time of 9 hours, 53 minutes, and 16 seconds, breaking the age record of Scottish Marathoner Jerry Wood-Allen, a ninety-year-old who completed the London Marathon.

Who is this champion and what can we learn from her? Gladys is the youngest of six children of Finnish immigrants. At age eleven she contracted polio but later recovered. The mother of five, Burrill lost her son Kevin to a brain tumor. Then, just two years before achieving the world record, her husband passed away. "I had a lot of obstacles in life," Gladys said, "but God was always there with me."[32] Adventure and exercise have also helped her deal with stress and grief throughout her life. In addition to her distance training, Burrill has been an airplane pilot and mountain climber.

I share Gladys's story because she is one of the All-Stars of Longevity—a person who has modeled CREATION Health living. Jim Barahal, president of the Honolulu Marathon, said he was astonished by Burrill's feat. "I think it is absolutely unbelievable," Barahal told KITV News. ". . . to realize what she is doing at her age. It is just astonishing. What an inspiration."[33]

Gladys's gift for inspiring others doesn't stop with exercise and adventure. She also gives of herself to help those in need and encourages others to do the same. According to news reports, Barahal and marathon organizers gave $2,500—in honor of Gladys—to the Lokahi Giving Project, which helps families in need with food and other basic necessities. Gladys says she does her best to use her local celebrity to help such projects. "I know what it's like to go through poverty," she says.

Gladys's words reveal the resilient spirit that caused the media to dub her the "Glady-ator." Her philosophy is that life is like a marathon, requiring perseverance, strength, and courage. "Sometimes I go out [walking] with the weight of the world on my shoulders and come back feeling so strong and renewed," Gladys says. "It's very important to think positive . . . dream about things you want to do in the future, even if they're impossible. It keeps you going."[34]

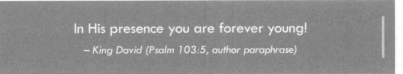

In His presence you are forever young!
— King David (Psalm 103:5, author paraphrase)

One mystery remains: why did she stop so close to the finish line? Her time could have been a full two minutes faster had it not been for the pause. Gladys explained that a few hundred feet from the finish line she stopped in order to pray, because in her words, "I thought my life would change once I crossed that line. I knew some people needed encouragement, so I thought that was very important!"[35] Remarkable! In the midst of her world record performance, Gladys paused to rest, pray, and trust in God—the source of her positive outlook and active life.

Gladys is also intent on passing on the legacy of CREATION Health to her eighteen grandchildren and twenty-six great grandchildren. Knowing that activity is a continual journey, not a destination, she regularly walks thirty to fifty miles a week, frequently accompanied by a training partner. Inspiration indeed!

THE REAL FOUNTAIN OF YOUTH

Is there a *real* source of eternal youth in this world? Not that we know of. But many researchers believe they have found the closest resource we have for staying young—physical activity that energizes the body, invigorates the mind, and refreshes the spirit. When physically challenged through regular exercise, the human body grows stronger and healthier and ages more slowly. In fact, regular activity benefits the whole person, including great gains for the mind, body, and spirit.

Sadly, according to the US Preventive Services Task Force, more than 70 percent of the population in the United States is not physically active. In fact, inactivity is said to be one of the greatest public health challenges of this century. Recent findings suggest that the incidence of stroke and type 2 diabetes would be lower, high blood pressure could be prevented or reduced, and bone fractures would occur less often if America just *moved* more. Many doctors are quick to admit that exercise is job one. There are no magic bullets in medicine, but the closest one is physical activity. People who are physically active cut their risk of heart disease in half.[36]

Research shows that regular physical exercise assists with the delivery of blood, oxygen, and nutrients to the brain. With regular activity the body sleeps better and is less susceptible to injury. Mentally, the body handles stress more effectively, the mind is able to think more clearly, and a person generally has a more positive outlook on life.

Socially, people often gain more confidence because they feel and look better. And spiritually, those who exercise often find a deeper connection to their Creator, who made them for a life of health, happiness, and peace. In short, active people are more alert, energetic, fun, caring, and alive! So why not make the choice to find time for physical activity on a consistent basis?

EDEN'S ACTIVITY

Activity is an important part of the CREATION Health model and a vital component of wholeness. This principle goes right back to the Garden of Eden.

The original paradise was indeed a beautiful, tranquil place. But contrary to some stereotypes, Adam and Eve didn't lie on a riverbank all day drinking fresh coconut juice. They didn't simply lounge around admiring pretty flowers and birds. While God *could* have designed their lives to be quite labor-free and passive, he had something else in mind.

"The Lord God took the man and put him in the Garden of Eden to work it and take care of it" (Genesis 2:15). Paradise, for Adam and Eve, wasn't a world of idleness. They were responsible for cultivating the garden and naming the animals. It was God's way of keeping them physically active.

Activity is how we experience the power of life. Great things happen when the mind, body, and spirit fully engage and reach a pinnacle. Athletes call it being in "the zone," actors give Oscar-level performances, artists create masterpieces, and authors pen award-winning works.

EXERCISE AND THE MIND

A founding principle of the Adventist Health System is an active lifestyle that stimulates the body, cultivates the mind, and inspires the spirit. Dr. John Harvey Kellogg, founding medical director of the Adventist Health System,[37] tested the strength of each patient and prescribed a personal exercise regimen for each one, including surgical patients—which was revolutionary. In the 1860s if you were suffering from heart disease, most physicians prescribed six weeks of total bed rest. Not Dr. Kellogg—he believed that exercise would speed healing, which is why he was one of the first to walk patients after surgery.

> A vigorous five-mile walk will do more good for an unhappy but otherwise healthy adult than all the medicine and psychology in the world.
> — Paul Dudley White

Dr. Kellogg invented and developed some of the first exercise equipment ever used, including the dynamometer (a muscle measurement device that was adopted by military academies), the stationary bicycle, the mechanical horse, and the rowing machine, among many others. His hospital included the first medical gymnasium, which was a model for modern fitness centers. Dr. Kellogg especially recommended walking, cycling, and swimming. He rode his own bicycle till he was ninety. To make exercise more fun he set it to music. Columbia Records sold a set of ten records that featured "A Scientific System of Exercise that builds the body's twenty-five major muscle groups."

In his book *The Living Temple* Dr. Kellogg asserted that, "Exercise quickens the stream of life, increases the action of the heart, lungs, stomach, liver, and every vital organ; and . . . so is one of the greatest of all means of promoting life and health. All examples of extraordinary longevity which have been reported have been of persons . . . whose habits in diet and in other respects were simple and regular."[38]

Physical activity affects more than just our bodies. It also helps our minds. Our body's organs are intricately interrelated. Everything inside us influences everything else. The state of our lungs affects the condition of our hearts. Our stomachs affect our intestines. Beyond that, our bodies can sway our minds. Perhaps you've heard about how our mental outlook or our level of stress can impact our physical health. Well, that's a two-way street. Mind affects body. But body also affects mind. Regular exercise can improve the overall attitude of our minds. In fact, exercise has a variety of psychological effects that enhance physical health. It buffers against stress, is an effective treatment for anxiety, and according to some researchers is as effective as psychotherapy in treating mild depression.[39] More good news, exercise can reduce the speed of aging.

LIVING BETTER, LIVING LONGER

Do you know the four leading causes today of preventable death and disability? They are cardiovascular disease (heart disease and stroke), cancer, diabetes, and lung disease. Many of these diseases are tied to lifestyle choices. According to an article published in the *Archives of Internal Medicine*, four lifestyle choices are considered cornerstones to a longer and better life: not smoking, maintaining a healthy weight, eating a wide variety of fruits and vegetables daily, and exercising regularly. Unfortunately the number of people engaging in all four healthy habits was a mere 3 percent![40]

The vast majority of Americans are not active on a regular basis—in spite of all the studies promoting the benefits of exercise. The Centers for Disease Control describes the problem this way: "American society has become 'obesogenic,' characterized by environments that promote increased food intake, nonhealthful foods, and physical inactivity."[41]

In the hospital we see the sad, catastrophic results of sedentary lifestyles, and we also witness the remarkable benefits of physical fitness. Simply walking thirty to forty minutes three to five times a week can diminish the risk of premature death from cancer and cardiovascular disease by 20 to 40 percent![42] Walking also has been shown to improve memory and to help prevent Alzheimer's.[43]

Many health experts believe that physical activity can truly be considered the wonder drug, because it strengthens the body to fight disease. In fact, purposeful activity may be the best medicine for fighting almost any disease. It helps the body battle stress, anxiety, and depression. It enables you to sleep better, look better, and feel better.

If you are in midlife your personal commitment to being physically active is critical. If you're not fit in your fifties, your projected life span is eight years less than if you are fit. Dr. Jarett Barry, a cardiologist at University of Texas Southwestern Medical Center in Dallas, presented this finding to the Heart Association Conference based on his study of 1,765 men and women. The research revealed that if you are fit in your fifties you double your chance of living to eighty-five.[44] So if you're approaching midlife, or even in your fifties, now is the time to get active and live active.

A fit life involves three different kinds of physical activity.

THREE KINDS OF PHYSICAL ACTIVITY

Three important kinds of physical activity are endurance, strength, and flexibility.

Endurance
Endurance activities involve cardiovascular or aerobic training. Such exercises work the heart and lungs, causing them to become

stronger and more efficient. Endurance exercise elevates the heart rate for a sustained period of time. This type of exercise is especially important for people who spend most of their day on a job that doesn't require much physical exertion. When you train your heart through endurance exercise one of the main benefits is that you will have more energy.

Whether running, walking, cycling, rowing, swimming, or doing any movement that gets your heart and lungs working, the results are multiple and valuable. Cardiovascular training is known to reduce the risk of heart disease, improve blood cholesterol and triglyceride levels, improve heart function, reduce the risk of osteoporosis, and improve muscle mass.[45] Endurance exercise is also important for weight management.

In the book *Creation Health Breakthrough*, Dr. Reed advises, "Your workout should be intense enough and long enough to achieve a cardiovascular training effect. Shoot for about thirty minutes, at least three times per week . . . . If you are trying to lose weight, try to work your way up to sixty minutes most days of the week. Start slowly and gradually work your way up. The intensity of your exercise should be strenuous enough that you feel you are working, but it doesn't need to be exhausting. If it is, you are less likely to stick with it."[46]

Dr. Reed also notes that you should always get your doctor's approval before starting an exercise program, especially if you are severely overweight, over age fifty, or suffer from a chronic disease like heart disease or diabetes.

Strength

Today there is increasing evidence about the value of strength training—which some call the best anti-aging weapon we have. It can benefit muscle mass, body fat percentage, blood-sugar tolerance, blood pressure, and bone density. A high muscle-to-fat ratio causes your metabolic rate—the rate at which you burn calories—to increase, making weight loss and weight management easier. Strong muscles also improve physical performance in whatever you're doing while also protecting against injury.

Experts increasingly emphasize that strength training is not only for the young. Its benefits can protect against the onset or reduce the symptoms of arthritis, diabetes, osteoporosis, and back pain. Strong muscles and bones reduce the likelihood and effect of falls. In fact, it may be more important to push yourself at strength training as you age.

Dr. Reed recommends strength training at least twice a week. "A basic program would include exercises using the major muscle groups of the arms, legs, and your body's 'core:' the shoulders, chest, abdomen, hips, pelvis, and the upper to lower back muscles . . . . Work your way to ten to twelve repetitions of the same exercise, take a brief rest, then repeat another set. Typically two sets are sufficient."[47]

One thing that's important to remember is that *all* our bodily functions start declining when our muscles weaken. So be sure to include regular strength training as part of your activity plan.

Flexibility

A third component of overall physical fitness is flexibility. Another problem with our modern sedentary lifestyle is that inactive muscles become stiff and more at risk to injury. That makes flexibility a crucial part of physical conditioning, especially as we age. When you are active and challenging your muscles, a stretching process takes place that adds flexibility and strength, making injury less likely.

Stretching isn't only for athletes. Stretching improves flexibility and range of motion, protects against injury, improves circulation, and relieves stress. You can stretch almost anytime or anywhere.

Many books and other resources are available that can give you good stretching exercises. But before starting any stretching routine, remember that inactivity causes muscles to stiffen—raising the possibility of injury. So make sure you start slowly when striving to increase your flexibility. Dr. Reed says, "It's important to warm up before stretching. Warming up will decrease stiffness and increase your range of motion while you stretch . . . . Stretching should feel good. Make sure you're stretching through the muscle's full range of movement until you feel a gentle resistance (not pain), then hold the maximum position for thirty to sixty seconds and relax. Don't bounce. Breathe freely."[48]

Dr. Reed also suggests engaging in a stretching routine at least three times a week for maximum benefit.

THREE MOTIVATIONS FOR ACTIVITY

Motivation and consistency are two of the challenges we face when it comes to maintaining a fitness plan. In the process of interviewing hundreds of active members (4,500 total members) at the Celebration Health Fitness Center I have found three motivators that keep them on the road to health.

First is the "me motivation," or participating in an activity for the purpose of improving myself. These people have a personal goal, and they are tenacious in pursuing it. They set specific goals for weight, strength, and diet, follow well-defined programs, chart their progress, and seldom miss a workout. They are so focused that they arrive at the gym, plug in their personal music player, and become so focused that they are almost oblivious to others around them. They go about their workout with the discipline of a pro athlete.

The second is the "we motivation." Here you find one or more friends to run together, walk together, or work out together. The effort is more about *us* than *me*. We have fun, encourage each other, and direct each other toward varied activities and sports. The benefits are both deeper friendships and physical fitness.

The third is the "they motivation." Now you are exercising and socializing for a cause, enhancing the experience with generosity and greater purpose. You take care of your body, encourage your friends, and improve your world.

Samantha, a business leader, wife, and busy mother of two wanted to improve her health. Since she's a social person, she challenged some friends to train with her to run the Disney half-marathon, which she'd never done before. As she and her friends got started, she got an idea. She told her friends, "You know, what would be even better than running the race would be running the race to make a difference for children!" They decided to seek sponsors and raise money for the Walt Disney Pavilion at Florida Hospital for Children. The idea was so energizing that more friends joined the effort, and eventually seventeen women crossed the finish line, having raised nearly $20,000.

The story doesn't end there. This group has become a magnet for more people wanting to join and train for future races. The enthusiasm has gone far beyond the physical benefits of running, to the gratification that they are doing something to make the world a better place. That's the multiplier effect of this dimension of activity. So if you're looking to motivate your friends to exercise—try fitness for a cause. It is a great place to start. Just ask Sam.

ACTIVITY IS A KEY TO MANAGING DISEASE

Jimm Bunch had practiced the 8 Secrets for most of his thirty-three years. He was a vegetarian and physically active. While attending UCLA where he anticipated receiving his MBA within three months, he received some shocking news. He was about to embark on his second cross-country bike trip with his soon-to-be wife when he learned he had type 1 diabetes—commonly known as "juvenile diabetes" because it normally appears during the teenage years or younger. He immediately started to wonder if he would ever be able to cycle cross country again.

"I didn't know anything about diabetes before I got it," Jimm says. "Of course, my initial reaction was worry and anxiety. But I knew I couldn't stay there. So I educated myself on how to manage the condition. I decided I wouldn't let it slow me down, and for the most part, it doesn't." Today Jimm is President of Park Ridge Hospital in North Carolina. Since his diagnosis he's been on two more cross-country bike trips.

Jimm says he has to stay in shape to keep up with his two sons who love skiing, hiking, and other outdoor activities. "Quite honestly, instead of limiting me, having diabetes has pushed me to pay more attention to living the way I want to live in the first place. It's almost an excuse to take excellent care of myself."

Jimm doesn't dwell on any negative aspects of his disease. In fact, when he's filling out routine medical forms, he often has to stop and remind himself that he's diabetic. The keys for him are his relationship with God, his family, and daily balance in food and activity.

"Next to the gene that causes diabetes is the gene that causes apathy," Jimm says with a wry smile. "There are a lot of doctors who don't like working with diabetics because so many of them don't try to control the condition. But I feel fortunate that of all the diseases I could have gotten, I have one that's manageable. I know the choices I make every day help determine my health destiny."

Jimm understands that as he is gets older, the CREATION Health principles are even more important. "I tell people to do something active every day. Just move! Even if it's only walking for a half hour. I know it works because I have to monitor my blood sugar constantly, and I can tell you, activity makes a difference."

So wherever you find yourself today, you can choose to engage in the active life that God intended for you. You can embrace and use your energy and abilities to nourish your spirit. Take a fresh approach to your daily activity. Engage life with purpose and meaning. This is what propels you toward a Healthy 100.

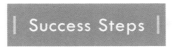

Success Steps

- **The Three Motivations** – Of the three motivations of activity— me, we, they—which would provide you with the most satisfaction? What step could you take today to engage in that motivation of activity?

- **Assess** – Use an "x" to mark your current level of physical activity on the scale below:

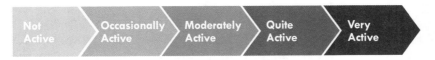

Now use an "o" to mark the level of activity you want to have one month from now. Use a capital "O" with a dot in the middle (i.e. a target) to indicate the level of activity you would aim to have a year from now.

- **Overcoming** – Which of the following seem to hinder your involvement in a more active lifestyle? And what can you do to overcome each one?

_____ Lack of time

_____ Lack of access to a place to exercise

_____ Lack of motivation

_____ TV and/or the Internet

_____ Lack of someone to exercise with

_____ Lack of appropriate attire and/or equipment

_____ Lack of energy

_____ The weather (or general climate)

• **Direction** – Keeping in mind that "activity is not a destination but a continual journey," what could you do to head in a better direction toward the goal of healthier, more active living . . .

Today: _____

This week: _____

This month: _____

The rest of this year: _____

• **Activity** – What can you do to increase your activity in the areas of . . .

Endurance: _____

Strength: _____

Flexibility: _____

8

TRUST

Why Trust is the Most Powerful Health Tool of All

A T THE BIRTH OF THEIR SECOND CHILD, TOM and Linda Starnes stood at the crossroads of life and death. Mac, their precious baby boy, would probably not live to see his first birthday. In that difficult moment they chose to put their trust in God as never before. Linda described their drama of faith:

> The day before Mac's birth, our obstetrician determined that Mac was in grave distress and might not make it through the birth process. But make it he did, gave one small cry, and was whisked away by a group of doctors and nurses.
>
> Weeks later after thirty surgeries or procedures under anesthesia, the physicians determined that Mac had "congenital bilateral perisylvian syndrome," such a rare syndrome that less than twenty cases had been diagnosed around the world. Mac was now the youngest to ever be identified.
>
> The best medical minds predicted that Mac would probably not live to see his first birthday, he would never learn to walk or talk, nor would he know us or have any "quality of life." We were given the choice to place a

"do not resuscitate" order on Mac or to place him on a ventilator to keep him alive.

Through many tearful prayers we made the best decision we could. Only God could make a decision about life for our little one—not us. We chose the following text as the motto for his life: "I will give thanks to You, for I am fearfully and wonderfully made; Wonderful are Your works, and my soul knows it very well" (Psalm 139:14). Leaving his life in God's hands, we asked that Mac be placed on a ventilator, and we made plans to spend Christmas at the hospital.

> Belief in God is the basis of all health.
> — John Harvey Kellogg, MD

We opened gifts, sang carols, and read a child's version of the Christmas story as a family. We also visited with Mac's "roommates" whose families were unable to be there.

It was a blessed Christmas day, difficult and teary at times, but we were joyful to be together as a family to honor another special Baby born so many years ago who came to save Mac, us, and the world.

It has been fifteen years since our most memorable Christmas. Our son defied all the doctors' predictions and the odds against him. Although he still has a trach and NG tube, uses technology and sign language to communicate, and has a bit of an unsteady gait, Mac is all boy. He is fully included with his peers at Lake Mary High School, is a percussionist with the marching band with his sister, and with a lot of hard work he maintains a "B" average. Mac has earned a third degree black belt in taekwondo, after a four-hour testing with a host of other students.

But most important, Mac is a happy, positive young man who made his own decision to come to Christ when he was six years old. Several years later he asked to be baptized, and so he was baptized in our family pool—trach and all!

Recently Mac was interviewed for a newspaper story. He answered the questions through his assistive technology device. When asked what he hoped to do after high school, Mac replied, "I want to be a pastor who travels around the world and spreads the word of God."

When asked what he would say to encourage others like him, Mac said, "God will be with you always, even in the hard times."

How blessed we have been to have him as a part of our family. We feel the world is all the better for his being here.

Tom and Linda's trust in God has had a national impact. Because of their passionate advocacy for the disabled they have helped to shape government policy. Linda was appointed by two presidents—Bush and Obama—to sit on the President's Committee for People with Intellectual Disabilities, serving as co-chair her final two years. Linda and Tom have helped found Access Ministries, an inclusive ministry for persons with disabilities and their families, first at their home church in Virginia, and then at their current church in Florida. In remembrance of their first Christmas in the hospital with Mac, Linda and her family join with Nathaniel's Hope every year to sing Christmas carols at the Walt Disney Pavilion Florida Hospital for Children and other area hospitals.

THE TRUST – HEALTH CONNECTION

Every day Mac demonstrates the relationship between healing and trust in God. But what effect does trust in God have on health? Dr. Jeff Levin's book *God, Faith, and Health* is one of the most thoroughly researched responses to this question. He has summarized over two hundred research studies published in peer review journals and identifies the following health benefits:

• Those with religious affiliations have a lower incidence of illness for the three leading causes of death in the US—heart disease, cancer, and hypertension.

• Regular church attendees have lower rates of illness and death than infrequent or non-attendees.

• Religiously active people live longer. Older people, in particular, enjoy a more active, less disabled life, with less depression and dementia than non-active persons. [49]

National Geographic highlighted faith in God as a key to increased longevity among Adventists.[50] Levin extends that finding to faith communities around the world. He identifies three overarching benefits of church membership:

1. Church membership benefits health by promoting healthy behavior and lifestyles.

2. Fellowship offers support that buffers the effects of stress and isolation.

3. Simple faith benefits health by leading to thoughts of hope, optimism, and positive expectation.

Trust in God provides strength for the "bad times" when disease and difficulty threaten your life while maximizing God's plan for your health in good times.

THE FOUNDATION OF ALL HEALTH

In his early writing Dr. John Harvey Kellogg stated, "Belief in God is the basis of all health." This bold assertion expresses the trust that the pioneers of the 8 Secrets placed in God as the source of health and healing. As a result, they developed a philosophy of health that encompassed the whole person—mind, body, and spirit. That is why the 8 Secrets, taken together, comprise a lifestyle as opposed to simply a diet or exercise program. Instead of the "spiritual" component serving as a desirable afterthought in relation to healthy living, it was recognized by Dr. Kellogg as the very foundation of all health. Every principle is intended to be experienced in mind, body, and spirit. You cannot be truly healthy if you have a fit body but suffer from a distressed mind or a depressed spirit.

> The best proof of love is trust.
> — Dr. Joyce Brothers

This vision of whole person health powered Dr. Kellogg and the other medical professionals who established the Adventist Health System. They trusted God and risked their careers, their finances, and their future on his design for healthy living.

TRUST IS AT THE CENTER OF LIFE

Trust is central to every relationship in life. That is the way that God designed the garden. At the center were two trees—the tree of life and the tree of knowledge of good and evil, providing Adam and Eve equal access to trusting God or trusting their own understanding. He did not hide the evil choice for it would have been unfair and manipulating to do so. Evil had equal opportunity to win human trust. He did not give the tree a repulsive name like the "tree of death." He did not force Adam and Eve to trust him. That would not have been loving. For trust to be loving it must be freely given; it cannot be forced. Trust is the most powerful tool you possess in relation to determining your health and happiness because it drives your choices. So make sure that what you trust and who you trust are worthy of your trust.

CHIEF OF THE MEDICAL STAFF

When Dr. John Guarneri became president of the medical staff he inaugurated the first physician-led Department of Spirituality and Health in a US Hospital. I have known Dr. Guarneri for a number of years, but I wanted him to tell me about the journey that led to his passion for integrating faith and medicine.

"When I started practicing medicine," Dr. Guarneri said, "like most newly minted physicians I was focused on caring for the physical needs of my patients: diagnosing, treating, educating. But over time many of the issues that I was dealing with had deeper root causes that could be traced to the patients' relationships. In order to go beyond simply treating symptoms to healing the patients' illnesses, I needed to invite patients to share these issues. I began to read the literature on spirituality and health and found that about 80 percent of patients wanted their physicians to discuss spiritual issues with them, but only 10 percent of the physicians actually did so. Initially, I was one of the doctors who had skirted the spiritual, largely because I didn't want to seem pushy or cross over into areas I didn't know how to handle. It was simply safer to confine myself to the realm of the physical. I decided that, while my training had provided me with the skills for caring for the body, I had not developed skills for listening to the mind and spirit of my patients.

"My journey to practice spiritual care began when I decided to ask one of my patients a simple question, 'Is there something in your life that is raising your stress level?'

'Yes, my husband and I have separated, and he has filed for divorce.'

'Would you like to talk about it?'" I asked.

"The conversation flowed, and I found myself recommending a good social support system and network. Since the patient was part of a faith community, I suggested a spiritual counselor and concluded by asking her if she would like to pray before she left. Suddenly I felt the awareness that the prescription that I had handed her was only part of the care that I could provide and that the prayer that we shared was healing for both of us! I sensed a profound moment of 'real healing.' I realized my calling to *extend the healing ministry of Christ.* I understood why Jesus went beyond physical healing in the lives of many of his patients. One of his patient encounters illustrates this. After healing a woman he concludes the encounter with the words 'your faith has made you whole.'

> Trust in the Lord with all your heart
> and lean not on your own understanding.
> — *Proverbs 3:5*

"The next few years I refined the spiritual healing dimensions of my practice. It became a passion for me. When I became the chief of the Florida Hospital Medical Staff, I wanted to advance our care in treating the whole person. The Medical Executive Committee embraced this idea, and we established the first physician-driven Department of Healthcare and Spirituality. What makes it so unique is that it is a clinical department that is physician driven but given equal standing to such medical disciplines as cardiology, oncology, orthopedics, and the like. It is led by physicians to provide a place where we recognize that trust in God is a path to health and healing.

PRAYER AND TRUST

The best way I can think of to express the importance of a personal life of prayer on health is to tell you about my friend Linda Nordyke Hambleton. At age six she was diagnosed with type I diabetes, and doctors did not expect her to live past age twenty-five. She outlived their predictions by more than twenty years, all the while waging an incredible battle for life that took her through 168 hospitalizations, two organ transplants, three cardiac arrests, three strokes, three years of blindness, and 250 grand mal seizures. While Linda's body was weakening under the burden of disease, her faith was strengthening under the blessing of prayer. Doctors told her she would never live to get married, but she married her childhood sweetheart Greg Hambleton.

> You trust and believe in people or life becomes impossible.
> — *Anton Chekhov*

At a number of community programs, Mary Lou and I interviewed Linda, her husband Greg, and her parents Karl and Bonnie Nordyke. Her faith so moved audiences that we asked her to write a book (*If Today Is All I Have*) that would describe her faith journey. The following excerpts from her book describe how her prayer life matured through the ups and downs of her disease. They are also my model for how to trust God in life and at death:

When the core of our being is threatened, that's when we find out that trust is not something you have; trust is something that you do moment by moment. Trust is a continual ongoing decision in the face of trying circumstances; it is a choice to believe in God's goodness and presence even when he seems to be steering our lives down the wrong path . . . .

During Linda's three-year experience with blindness, she found comfort by going to her prayer closet—not a figurative spot of solitude, but a literal prayer closet. With the world all around shrouded in darkness, Linda found great comfort sitting in her small closet where she could reach out and touch all four walls . . . where she knew no one could hear her as she prayed aloud. It became a personal place of intimacy and openness with God.

After Linda completed multiple surgeries that finally restored some of her eyesight, she continued to go to her closet to pray. She felt drawn to return to this solitary space where she shared intimacy with God. Linda's prayers often began with whys—Why blindness? Why diabetes? Why me? Why now? But over time they took on a different tone:

I finally made a transition between the "why" question to making a conscious and deliberate choice to trust the God that I loved. The focus of my heart changed from the discouraging and depressing circumstances around me to what I knew to be true about God himself. Nothing had changed outwardly, but the anger and frustration began to dissipate. While sitting in the closet I had taken a small step and discovered that the smallest mustard seed of faith can move mountains of confusion and conflict from the human heart. Where anger had been, God began to build something different: a heart of thanksgiving.

By an act of my will, with that small amount of faith, I was able to talk to him about the obvious good around me. Then I began to thank him for the things that I could see no good in whatsoever. God honored that small seed of faith, and when it was watered with my thanksgiving, it began to grow into something else: peace. As the bumper sticker says, "No God, No Peace. Know God, Know Peace." By finding him, I found the peace, and that's really what I had been looking for all along.

God was using the pain, suffering, and injustice of worldly life to continually draw me back into the closet where I could meet him . . . . So many questions have yet to be answered. So many tears continue to be shed. But as King David admitted to God in one of his closet poems, "You keep track of all my sorrows. You have collected all my tears in your bottle. You have recorded each one in your book" (Psalm 56:8). What did he find? He found that God was close enough to capture his tears in a bottle. To be that close, to be able to catch our tears, means God must be right here, eye to eye, touching our cheek. And when we are face down in despair, God takes the same posture, sharing our grief with us.

Finally, Linda describes her prayer response to the moment when medicine could do no more:

There is nothing left for us to do. I've been here before, of course, at the crossroads of faith and despair. That place where darkness seems impenetrable, where pain clouds everything and the future is so undefined, so vague and so full of fear. Yes, I've been here before, and I know where to go. It's closet time again. Time to let it all out, raise the fist of frustration, release tears of despair, and talk friend-to-friend with the only One who does know. Through the darkness—one more time, until I discover it—one more time.[52]

> Where is God when it hurts? He is in you, the one hurting; not in it, the thing that hurts.[51]
>
> — Dr. Paul Brand

I had the privilege of presenting Linda's eulogy, and I chose to read excerpts from her closet prayers. Linda exemplified living the spirit of a Healthy 100 even if her physical condition prevented attaining the chronological age. In the end it was not the pain that defined Linda's life, but her prayers. No one relished good health more than Linda—when it flashed across the darkness of her life she was the first to declare the goodness of God. She also knew the prayers of struggle and surrender, fear and faith, trepidation and trust. May it be true for you. In your moment of darkness, may prayer be the path that leads you through to the light of God's love.

Success Steps

- **Grow Trust** – Do you need Linda's kind of trust in your own life? To read more of Linda's inspiring story, seek out her book *If Today Is All I Have: Finding the Light of Hope in Dark Places* (for more information see FloridaHospitalPublishing.com). You can also learn more about Linda by visiting Healthy100.org/Linda.

- **Use Adversity as a Platform for Encouraging Others** – Mac's story of overcoming disability by using it as a platform to share his faith with others is truly inspiring. Though you are likely not as "disabled" as Mac, all of us are "disabled" to some degree, since none of us is perfectly whole. Identify your own most significant disability, and then generate a list of three things you could do to use it as a means of encouraging others.

- **Attend Church Regularly** – If you attend church regularly, what health-related benefits do you experience as a result? If you don't attend church, would improving your health (including your spiritual health, of course) be a good reason to make a change?

- **Ask yourself** – "If today is all I have" and I knew that for a fact, how would I live today?

9

INTERPERSONAL

*Love is Only Realized
in Relationship*

PERFORMING DELICATE HEART SURGERY UNDER the best conditions is a challenge, but in the middle of a war zone, a medical team needs extra supplies of courage, focus, and conviction. In 1974 Dr. Elsworth Wareham and a heart surgery team from California's Loma Linda University risked their lives in war-ravaged Saigon. These pioneers performed the first open-heart surgery in Vietnam, and over the course of nineteen operating days completed more than sixty lifesaving procedures.

Dr. Wareham and a senior medical student, Roger Hadley, had operated on a fourteen-year-old girl, Mi Thi. They intended to return to Vietnam to check on her progress one year later, but the fall of Saigon on April 30, 1975, halted that idea. However, thirty-five years later, Dr. Roger Hadley (who by this time had become dean of the Loma Linda University School of Medicine) received this e-mail: "My mother was operated on by a group of American doctors in April 1974 (in Saigon) and she's trying to find her surgeons." After a few more e-mails and pictures, Mi Thi confirmed that Dr. Hadley assisted Dr. Wareham in performing her surgery. She recounted a heroic journey from concentration camps to refugee camps to "boat person" status, finally finding her way to Canada where she married a French Canadian, adopted a new name, Wynn, and had two children.

At the invitation of Wynn, Drs. Hadley and Wareham flew to Victoria to celebrate the power of love to transform lives. Wynn said, "It was more exciting than my wedding day."

In the course of his career Dr. Wareham has performed more than 12,000 open heart surgeries a phenomenal record, been the guest of two US presidents in the Oval Office, appeared on the Oprah Winfrey show, and been invited to palaces in Greece and Saudi Arabia, but he said that seeing Wynn was the "highlight of my life." How could one of

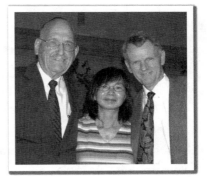

Dr. Elsworth Wareham, Mi Thi, Dr. Roger Hadley [Photo courtesy of Loma Linda University]

12,000 surgeries be more memorable than visiting with presidents and monarchs? Simple love is more rewarding than fame!

At ninety-four years of age, Dr. Wareham, a Longevity All-Star, was interviewed by Dr. Mehmet Oz for a television show on living longer and living better (Healthy100.org/Wareham). The TV crew followed Dr. Wareham as he assisted with open heart surgeries. Dr. Oz was so impressed with Dr. Wareham's vitality that he exclaimed, "He is my role model." Here is a man who traces his longevity to loving God and caring for others. I would suggest that he could be your role model as well.[53]

Giving yourself in service to others is at the core of creating and maintaining healthy interpersonal relationships. You have undoubtedly felt the internal satisfaction that comes from helping someone else—it is called the "helper's high." A generous life invested in helping others will boost your happiness and longevity.

Stephen Post, PhD, taught medical ethics at Case Western University Medical School for eighteen years before launching his research institute. In his book *Why Good Things Happen to Good People* he writes, "I have one simple message to offer and it's this: giving is the most potent force on the planet. Giving is the one kind of love you can count on, because you can always choose it: it's always within your power to give."[54] After years of studying this phenomenon, Post summarizes that giving protects overall health twice as much as aspirin protects against heart disease.[55]

A 1999 study led by Doug Oman of the University of California, Berkeley, found that elderly people who volunteered for two or more organizations were 44 percent less likely to die over a five-year period than were non-volunteers, even after controlling for their age, exercise habits, general health, and negative health habits like smoking.[56] In 2003 a University of Michigan study of seniors confirmed these findings.[57] The health impact of helping others is stronger than exercising four times a week and attending religious services. Stopping smoking is the only life change that is stronger than reaching out to meet the needs of others. Therefore, engaging in acts of generosity motivated by love for others is one of the strongest positive actions you can take to improve your health and positively affect your longevity.

GENEROSITY HEALS

Want to live longer? Love more. Psychiatrist Dr. Karl Menninger wrote, "Love cures—both the ones who give it and the ones who receive it."[58] If you are sick, generous love can speed your healing. Researchers have found that when you reach out to others, even when you are sick and may not feel like it, you release the positive endorphins that speed healing.

When Benji Watson was fourteen, he learned he had cancer. His family was devastated by this news, but Ben remembers thinking: *I am going to be a cancer survivor.* While courage and determination of this type definitely contribute to healing when one faces non-Hodgkins B-cell lymphoma and the various rounds of chemo and radiation treatment, Ben's mind was not focused on his disease. Instead he took notice of the other kids in the cancer ward. Ben soon learned that many of his fellow pediatric cancer fighters were not as blessed as he was by family, friends, school, and church. For example, many parents couldn't afford to take time off of work to stay with their kids. And there were many other needs as well.

Because of this, Ben asked if he could start a foundation to help pediatric cancer patients that had needs their families were unable to meet. With the help of his family, Ben formed the Benji Watson Cancer Foundation to help families of cancer-stricken kids pay for unexpected incidental costs while their children were hospitalized. The foundation's first event "The Benji Buzz Haircut"raised $11,000. But Ben didn't stop there. By the end of the summer, contributors had raised a total of $30,000—not bad for a fourteen-year-old cancer fighter. When asked about this extraordinary feat Ben simply says, "I give back because I know that generosity heals." If you would like to see a short video on Ben's story, visit Healthy100.org/Ben. Or, to find out more about The Benji Watson Cancer Foundation, visit BensVoice.org.

FRIENDS FOR LIFE

Tom Rath, author of the book *Vital Friends*, asserts, "Friendships are among the most fundamental of human needs. This is not simply a statement of personal conviction but it comes from years of Gallup research. The fact is, we are biologically predisposed to this need for relationships, and our environment accentuates this every day. Without friends, it is very difficult for us to get by, let alone thrive."[59]

Eugene Kennedy, PhD, professor of psychology at Loyola University of Chicago, says, "Friendship has a profound effect on your physical well-being. Having good relationships improves health and lifts depression."[60] Many studies back up this statement. One found that older individuals who perceived their social support as impaired were 340 percent more likely to die prematurely from all causes.[61]

Rath adds, "During our teenage years we spend nearly one-third of our time with friends. For the rest of our lives, the average time spent with friends is less than ten percent."[62] Perhaps this is why so many of our friendships can be traced back to high school. Recent studies have shown that behaviors such as happiness, obesity, smoking, and altruism are "contagious" within adult social networks. Research also points out that if your best friend eats healthily, you're five times more likely to also eat healthy. If your best friend exercises, you're 100 percent more likely to be active!

The University of Michigan researchers found that in women, friendships increase the hormone progesterone, which enhances a sense of well-being while reducing anxiety and stress.[63]

FRIENDS ENHANCE YOUR WORK PERFORMANCE

Gallup workplace research based on a national sample of 1,000 workers found that "people with at least three close friends at work are more likely to be extremely satisfied with their life."[64] Friendships are clearly vital to happiness and achievement on the job.

I was captivated by the application of this principle in a historic victory for the United States team in the 2008 Ryder Cup golf matchthe most prestigious team golf event in the world. Since the inception of the event, the US had amassed an impressive record of victories, bringing home the trophy twenty-two out of twenty-five matches between 1927 and 1983 (it was generally a biennial event). But after winning the matches in 1983 the US team had won only three times in twenty-five years. The pressure was mounting; national pride and global leadership were at stake. Hall of Fame golfer Paul Azinger, known to his friends as "Zinger," was chosen to captain the 2008 team. Sports writers and psychologists attributed the poor performance of the US to their inability to come together as a team. They pointed out that the US had the highest ranked golfers in the world, but the teamwork of the Europeans enabled them to dominate. Was the problem American independence, superstar egos, or lack of leadership? When Zinger was selected as team captain, I asked him how he planned to break this string of losses.

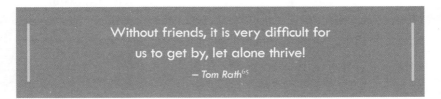

Without friends, it is very difficult for us to get by, let alone thrive!

— *Tom Rath*[65]

Paul's answer was so unusual and yet so effective that it was chronicled in the excellent book *Cracking the Code*. This book is based on an incredible golfing achievement, but the principles apply to any work setting where teamwork is vital to success. It is all about how to get different personalities to work together to achieve their best. Paul engaged his friend and relationship specialist, Psychologist Dr. Ron Braund, in the search for a winning strategy. Together they crafted a plan that would become the foundation for victory. I want to share three components of this plan with you:

• Break the twelve-man team into small pods of four players each;

• Select the members of the pods based on their personality types rather than particular strengths in their golf games;

• Have players practice in their pods versus alone.

The results—victory chant that echoed across the fairways of the Valhalla Golf Club signifying a historic victory. The chant burst into a national celebration as Captain Azinger led the American team onto the balcony for an uproarious and lengthy standing ovation. The victory was the most decisive since 1981—despite the absence of the number one player in the world due to injury. Zinger's comments to the press focused on the power of interpersonal relationships, "We were more than a team. We were a family." This band of friends, including spouses and children, will share this victory for years to come. But its greatest reward will eclipse the trophy, for that memory is now history, but their friendships are always present, current, and meaningful. The message: friendships win at home, at work, at play for all of life throughout all of eternity.

THE LONELINESS OF ONE AND THE LOVE OF TWO

Throughout the creation story the phrase "it was good" is repeated as God surveys his work with joyful satisfaction. Only one time in the story is this refrain broken and God says "it is not good." This dramatic dissonance in the story is no accident it does not occur as a celestial surprise. God's statement is meant to punctuate the human need for friendship and family. God has orchestrated the moment by creating Adam without a partner, while he created all of the animals in pairs of male and female. God gives Adam the privilege of naming the animals, and as they parade by in couples he becomes increasingly aware of his loneliness. As Adam's isolation peaks, God declares what Adam feels, "It is not good for man to be alone." By heightening Adam's awareness of his need for companionship, God prepared him to cherish Eve as a soul mate that he would never take for granted.

The first recorded words of man are Adam's commitment to Eve. In fact they are written in the form of a song . . . a wedding song that Adam sings, "Finally! Bone of my bone, flesh of my flesh! Name her Woman for she was made from Man. That is why a man leaves his father and mother and unites with his wife, and they become one flesh."

This moment is the high point of the sixth day of creation, for humans have been rescued from their deepest threat—isolation that breeds loneliness. Instead God gave them more—for it is through the love of a man and a woman that he created the bond of marriage and the birth of children.

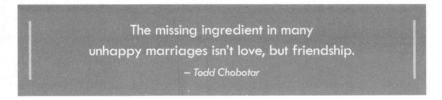

The missing ingredient in many unhappy marriages isn't love, but friendship.

— *Todd Chobotar*

Love is realized in relationship; God is three persons unified in one. The God of creation is not a solitary figure positioned high above humanity but a trinity of love walking in the garden among his creation seeking and celebrating relationship.

When the garden is lost and Jesus returns to a broken world, his first miracle occurs at a wedding. It is as though he is reenacting the wedding of Adam and Eve. His restoration of love is focused on the marriage of a man and a woman, and the tempo of eternity is reaffirmed.

HEALTH BENEFITS OF A HAPPY MARRIAGE

According to Gallup research, a couple's friendship accounts for

70 percent of overall marital satisfaction—"five times as important as physical intimacy."[66] In a great marriage, physical intimacy is a celebration of friendship. In a previous book I suggested that giving your spouse a massage while you talk about the day could be a great way to express your love. I received a thank-you letter from a couple who had been married for over forty years. They adopted the couples massage and said that they were enjoying a new level of intimacy that they had not experienced and only wished that they had begun it years earlier.

> Today we are faced with the pre-eminent fact that,
> if civilization is to survive,
> we must cultivate the science of human relationships.
>
> — President Franklin D. Roosevelt's last words

With that endorsement, I am again suggesting that your deepest moments of friendship occur when you are fully focused on the other person and their best good. Why? Because your spouse will sense the greatest affirmation—your full attention!

DEFINING LOVE AND FIGHTING FAIR

Mary Lou and I recently celebrated our forty-sixth wedding anniversary. Forty-five of those years have been happy. But that first year was stormy—it was the hurricane year of adjustment. After cooling down from a particularly volatile encounter, we realized that we could not allow this pattern to continue. If we wanted our marriage to last we had to come to an agreement on how we would solve our differences.

We decided two things: First, we would write our definition of love—the kind of love we wanted to realize through our relationship.

Second, we would agree on rules for fighting fair. These two steps have proved to be so valuable that when we provide premarital counseling to a couple, we ask them to do the same. We would also like to recommend these two steps to you. Listed below is the definition of love we wrote together:

Love is a plant that grows in the common ground of spiritual unity.
Watered by a spring of communication,
It blossoms in the sunlight of affection.

For years this definition occupied prime billboard space on our refrigerator. It reminded us to invest in spiritual unity, communication, and affection. We committed to making sure that whatever our differences might be we would follow the advice of Scripture: ". . . do not let the sun go down on your anger, and do not give the devil an opportunity" (Eph. 4:26–27, NASB). Our primary rule was to resolve our differences before they caused us to become distanced from each other—before we went to bed at night. That one rule assured that we rested in unity, not adversity. United, not divided.

THE SUNLIGHT OF AFFECTION

One of the hazards of marriage is that life becomes too routine, and routine lacks romance. Romance is spontaneous and delightfully surprising. It specializes in the joy of small tokens of affection at unexpected moments. It thrives in words of affirmation.

Longevity All-Stars retain romance throughout their lives. Listen to the words of Dr. Ernest Rogers who, at age ninety-five, describes how he fell in love with his new bride, Annell, age ninety-three: "Here is an angel of delight, and I must try to find an inroad into her loveliness." When you speak the language of love you are speaking the language of eternity, and it makes you feel forever young. God is the greatest romantic, and it is his love that keeps Dr. Rogers young and vibrant—and it will do the same for you.

The Rogers romance so captivated television producers that the couple was featured in a recent television PBS special titled "Over 90 and Loving It!" If you would like to view that video, please visit Healthy100.org/Rogers.

WHEN FRIENDSHIP FINDS A WAY

Friendships in the workplace can lead the culture of an organization when they rise above the divisive forces of competition that threaten to fracture unity. I had the rare privilege of seeing this principle in action. It was 1999 and Mardian Blair, president of the Adventist Health System, announced his retirement. The two leading candidates for this vital role were consummate professionals and close personal friends.

The competitive grapevine began to hum with the news, and the political tensions began to mount. It was apparent that this process could result in a win/lose environment that would not only affect their relationship but could create a divisive climate in the organization. Sensing the stakes, these two leader friends chose to write an open letter to the board. An excerpt from the letter provides you with a model of what it takes to be a friend:

> The society in which we live places great significance in being #1 and many of us find it easy to classify performance in terms of winning or losing, and individuals as winners or losers. It is unfortunate that more of us are not able to view events and people through the eyes of the apostle Paul who saw himself as a winner in the race, but not to the exclusion of others, but a winner in a race in which all who identify with Christ are winners.
>
> It is in this context that this letter is being written ... Both of us have the highest regard for each other from a professional perspective, and there is no other individual that we would rather see receive the appointment.

Equally important, and perhaps more importantly, we enjoy a personal friendship that is of great significance to us. We are not going to permit the outcome of the selection process to negatively impact that valued aspect of our lives. In many ways our relationship is similar to that of David and Jonathan who were close friends, both before and after one of them was named as king. It is our purpose to realize a similar outcome.

Just as the two of us view each other as winners today, we will view each other as winners after the selection is made . . . It is not about winning and losing, it is about doing God's work. It is our prayer that God will direct in the selection that is made for the CEO . . . as we work together to fulfill our mission of extending Christ's healing ministry.

Signed,
Donald L. Jernigan   *Thomas L. Werner*
Executive Vice President   *Executive Vice President*

Success Steps

Here are seven steps to get you started thinking about how to improve your interpersonal relationship success:

- **Give Yourself to Others** – While you may not have a chance to save someone's life or repair a defect surgically, the gift of yourself is the greatest gift you can give. Name three ways you could help someone else by giving of your time or talent or money or simply by giving them some encouragement.

- **Practice Generosity** – As Benji Watson says, "Generosity heals." There are many ways to live a life of generosity besides giving money. What do you have that you could give to make a difference in someone else's life?

- **Treasure and Protect Your Friendship** — Too often people take their friendships for granted and fail to nurture and strengthen them as much as possible. Write down the names of your three best friends and something you could do today to let each one know how important he/she is to you.

- **Commit to Teamwork at Home and at Work** — Ecclesiastes 4: 9–10 says, "Two are better than one, because they have a good return for their work: If one falls down, his friend can help him up. But pity the man who falls and has no one to help him up!" What could you do to become more of a team player, at home and at work?

- **Keep Your Romance Alive** — by loving your spouse creatively and spontaneously. Give him or her a massage and a listening ear. Delight yourself in your spouse, and keep falling in love, following Dr. Rogers's example, "Here is an angel of delight, and I must try to find an inroad into her loveliness."

- **Love Others Sacrifically** — Recall a time when your most constructive direction might have been to adopt an attitude like that exhibited by Don and Tom. What did you say or do? Was that choice easy or difficult to make? What might you say or do differently should a similar situation arise in the future?

10

OUTLOOK

Pursuing the Positive Power of Optimism and Hope

T HE MORNING BEGAN LIKE ANY OTHER, YET this morning would change her life. Sheila stepped into the shower, but something was different, unusual, unsettling. As she turned off the water and stepped out of the shower, she glanced into the mirror and the unsettled feeling changed to deep concern, because the shape of one of her breasts was noticeably different. As she performed a self-exam she found a lump. At age forty, she had not yet had her first mammography.

Being a woman of action, without delay she went to see her doctor. After a diagnostic mammogram Sheila was told she had stage four breast cancer, the recommended treatment for which is a mastectomy.

When the surgery was performed, the pathology report revealed that the cancer had invaded twenty-four of the thirty-one lymph nodes that had been removed. Devastated by the news, she and her husband, Tom, determined to attack the cancer with all of the resources they could muster—physical, mental, and spiritual.

Physically, Sheila embarked on an intense regime of chemotherapy followed by radiation. She then researched and adopted healthier lifestyle practices. Mentally, she researched the disease and the best ways to fight it. She read and analyzed information from many sources, including the most recent findings and the personal stories of many who had faced this disease.

She described her spiritual strategy, perhaps the most important factor of all:

The medical terms rang in my mind—"cancer," "stage four," "malignant lymph nodes," and all the rest. And when you hear words like those, the attack on your spirit can be as malignant as the attack on the body. I had no hope; in fact I was afraid to hope, because I didn't want to have my hopes dashed by death. But my immediate family (our four sons and Tom) and my church family surrounded me with support. My first lesson of healing was that you can borrow hope from people around you. They bring you promises, share prayers, and surround you with encouragement. So I borrowed their hope and began to rebuild my spirit.

I knew that I would lose my hair and wouldn't like what I saw in the mirror, so I decided to make my mirror a "marquee of hope." I used a permanent magic marker, because I didn't want the words to wash off, and I wrote words of hope across the same bathroom mirror that had first revealed the illness to me, words like peace, joy, overcomer, victor—many of which were hope gifts that others had given me.

As a result, when I looked in that mirror, I did not see a sick person waiting to die, but a person facing a difficult challenge with hope in her heart. It's important to remember that I didn't have to generate my own hope, especially at first. I borrowed it from others until, over time, it became my own.

I needed hope most at night. Night after night the 3 AM chemo alarm would shake me from my sleep—with one recurring question echoing in my mind: What will they do if I die? You see I had invested my life in my boys—Tommy, 13; Andrew and Sam, 12; and Noah, 7. I loved being their mother.

This haunting question was rooted in a poignant afternoon discussion with my seven-year-old. My hair had fallen out, my eyes had dark circles from the effects of chemo and sleep deprived nights, and from all outward appearances it looked like the cancer was winning. Noah sat down beside me. He took my face in his hands and looked deep into my eyes and asked, "Mommy, are you going to die?" Through faces bathed in tears we talked about our fears. Our hope seemed to be siphoned out of our hearts and was running down our cheeks.

Noah's question tormented me for several days. Finally, in the darkness of an early morning, after another sleepless night, I couldn't take it anymore. I didn't want to wake my husband, but I had to know, "Tom," I said, interrupting his sleep. "What are you going to do if I die?" He rolled over, wrapped his strong arms around me, and repeated for the third night in a row, "Sheila, I promise you I will take care of the boys and raise them just like we planned. But, I have been thinking about this question since you began asking me and I have a question for you." He paused, and I thought, What question could be more important than the one I just asked him? Then he asked me a question that completely spun me around. "Sheila," he said, "the real question is what are you going to do if you live?"

This question so affected Sheila's thought process that she completely altered her goal from being a cancer survivor to becoming a conqueror. Her favorite biblical text became, ". . . in all these things we are more than conquerors through him who loved us" (Romans 8:37). She began to think about the future and what she could do to take her life back from the disease that was stalking her. Her battle cry became: "No reserve. No regrets. No return. Full speed ahead." The next morning Sheila announced, "I know what I'm going to do. I'm going to pursue my dream of becoming a doctor. I'm going back to finish my pre-med studies at UCF (University of Central Florida)."

And so it happened that when she finished chemotherapy, she enrolled in her first course, neurobiology, because the research she had done on the effects of chemo indicated that it could impact the executive function of the brain. She entered with apprehension that she could compete with the bright young minds of her classmates, but in the end she finished at the top of the class. Throughout the two-year completion of her daunting pre-med science courses she compiled a GPA that placed her at the top of her class. Each time she aced a course she declared, "Take that, cancer!"

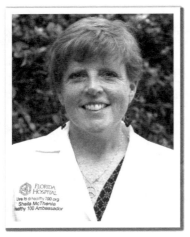

Sheila — The first Healthy 100 Ambassador [Photo by Meredith Tipton]

Three years passed. She completed her chemotherapy treatments and her pre-med studies while remaining symptom-free. Though Sheila and her doctors were not ready to declare that the cancer was cured, she was ready to declare how a changed outlook had changed her life. With the help of her family she was able to move from the helplessness of disease to the hopefulness of faith. Sheila's goal is to become a physician who focuses on preventing, detecting, and treating breast cancer among women who cannot afford care. For the record, she passed her MCAT—the test that students must pass to apply to medical school—with flying colors.

But then a new question surfaced. "Don't you think you're too old to become a doctor?" people would ask. Sheila's eyes would dance with delight when she would respond, "Not at all. I'm planning to live to a hundred, and that gives me a long time to practice medicine!" At the end of our interview Sheila summed up her outlook on life, "Only the Lord knows how long I will live, but he allows me to determine how intensely I will live each day." It is because Sheila has chosen to embrace this outlook on life that Florida Hospital honored her as the first Healthy 100 Ambassador.

IGNITED BY INSPIRATION

The presence of God in us is the source of our inspiration! Remember the sixth day of creation, when the Creator sculpted Adam's body from the earth, then breathed life into the man's nostrils. It was a miracle moment, as life-giving breath inflated Adam's lungs, activated his heart, stimulated his brain, and ignited his spirit, and Adam "became a living soul." This moment in history is known as the "inspiration of humanity," from the words "in spire" (to breathe into). To live "life to the full" is to be inspired. The opposite of inspired living is to have the breath of God leave you as you expire and die.

> Adopting the right attitude can convert
> a negative stress into a positive one.
> — Dr. Hans Selye

T. Denny Sanford, a friend whom I admire greatly, has a personal motto that I love: "Aspire to Inspire, Before you Expire." He has done just that through a remarkable life of philanthropy. What makes Denny such an exceptional person is that he possesses a brilliant mind for business and a passionate heart for people.

You were made for inspiration, the moments when your body, mind, and spirit are fully charged with life. You can live by respiration—simply breathing in the atmosphere around you. But the moment that you experience the "breath of God" filling you with love, you become creative, great thoughts fill your mind, great emotions ignite your spirit, and great actions flow from your body. When the "breath of God" sweeps across artists they see life in all its beauty and capture it in full detail, creating masterpieces. Musicians compose timeless songs that create memories. Poets write sonnets that time cannot erase. Orators craft thoughts into phrases that shape the sayings of generations to come. This is the power of inspiration. This is what excites us with living and makes moments eternal. Through inspiration God will gift you with a hopeful future and a positive present, which is why it is the place to start when you want to build a positive outlook.

This God-filled living gives hope to your daily life and work. It gives you the eyes to see goodness, the ears to hear goodness, and the actions to extend goodness. Isn't it interesting that the word "goodness" comes from "God ness," in other words, God-like-ness. You can live with hope in a broken world if you are inspired by God to create goodness wherever you can, to push back the boundaries of bad, and to realize that though you cannot fix everything, someday God will bring heaven to earth and replace all evil with goodness. So live with hope and act with goodness!

THE SCIENCE OF HOPE

John Harvey Kellogg, the first medical director of the Adventist Health System, said, "Hope is the most powerful stimulant for the body."

Our outlook on life has significant impact on our physical, mental, and spiritual health. We all have challenges and pitfalls. "True hope has no room for delusion," writes oncologist Jerome Groopman, MD, in *The Anatomy of Hope*. "Clear-eyed hope gives us the courage to confront our circumstances and the capacity to surmount them. For all my patients, hope, true hope, has proved as important as any medication."[67]

The opposite of hope is despair, which attacks our mind, body, and spirit. It knocks the breath of God out of our lungs of hope and does untold damage to our well-being. Despair often expresses itself as depression. A fifteen-year study done by Kaiser Permanente concluded that depressed people utilized healthcare services five times more than the normal population.

Dr. Richard Davidson at the University of Wisconsin discovered that people with a positive attitude have more electrical and metabolic activity on the left side of the brain's prefrontal lobe.[68] In one recent study researchers surveyed 2,432 older Canadians about their quality of life. Those who maintained excellent health over an entire decade were considered *thrivers*. "We found that people who had a positive outlook and lower stress levels were more likely to thrive in old age," said Mark Kaplan, lead author.[69]

> Hope is not a way out but a way through.
> — *Robert Frost*

THE IMPACT OF PESSIMISM AND DEPRESSION

Ongoing research shows what a tremendous influence depression has on all aspects of a person's life. "Depression jumps out as an independent risk factor for heart disease," reports Dwight Evans, professor of psychiatry, medicine, and neuroscience at the University of Pennsylvania. "It may be as bad as cholesterol."[70]

By contrast, hope gives birth to optimism, the natural antidepressant. So how can you acquire this outlook on life? An essential first step is to accept the fact that bad things will happen! They happen to everyone. But how you view the bad things that happen in your life (both large and small) can be a key shaping your outlook and improving your health. For example, what if you discovered that you'd lost your wallet and despite your best efforts you were unable to find it? Or what if your phone was to ring right now and the voice on the other end informed you that something terrible happened that will affect you for the rest of your life? How would you explain this problem to yourself? Which of the thoughts below would best represent your self-talk? Where would you place yourself on the line between the two thoughts?

This is bad.　　　　　　　　　　　　　　　　　　**This is bad.**
But it doesn't represent my life.　　　**It is the way my life works.**
It is only temporary.　　　　　　　　**I always end up getting hurt.**

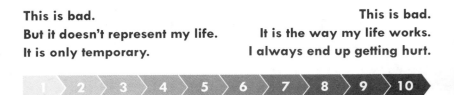

In his classic book *Learned Optimism,* Martin E.P. Seligman, PhD, looked for specific differences between optimists and pessimists. After twenty-five years of study, he wrote, "Whether or not we have hope depends on two dimensions of our explanatory style: pervasiveness and permanence."[71] Seligman found that the defining characteristic of pessimists is that they tend to believe bad events will last a long time (permanence), will undermine everything they do (pervasiveness), and are their own fault. They view life with *learned helplessness.* He believes that this persistent strain of pessimism—the belief that actions aimed at improving things will be futile—accounts for the upsurge of depression in this country.

"The optimists, who are confronted with the same hard knocks of the world, think about misfortune in the opposite way. They tend to believe defeat is just a temporary setback, that its causes are confined to this one case."[72] But hopelessness is not hopeless, so what are some strategies for building hope?

POSITIVITY RATIO

Dr. Barbara Fredrickson's research has revealed that a key to experiencing an optimistic outlook on life is the ratio of positive emotions to negative emotions. Optimists tend to have three positive emotions to one negative emotion. If you're not used to thinking this way, how might you experience this 3:1 ratio? She suggests that you learn to be open to the goodness around you. Goodness is plentiful. The problem is that we can be so focused on the negative that we fail to perceive the positive, and it passes by unnoticed.

Dr. Fredrickson even suggests scheduling "rest stops" in your day as a way to improve your ratio. In other words, if you will stop, look, and listen, you will begin to be aware of the beauty and goodness that is vital to lifting your spirits. Rest enhances outlook!

OUT WITH THE BAD –
IN WITH THE GOOD . . . EMOTIONS

In his book *Pain Free for Life*, Dr. Scott Brady describes his own experience of finding relief from severe pain through a process that involves the mind and spirit, as well as the body. He describes what amounted to an epiphany, "I understood the true cause of my pain—the strong, negative, repressed emotions—and that the pain could be cured by releasing and neutralizing those emotions . . . . Finally, I had my life back—without pain or pills. I could hit golf balls without throwing out my back, and I could deal with pressure-filled situations at home or work without getting a headache or a bout of irritable bowel."[73]

Resolving damaging emotions is a fundamental part of returning to health and speeding healing. Positive emotions have their greatest effect when we stop to celebrate them! Be a collector of the positive, scouting the landscape of life for goodness, and when you spot it, stop, set aside the cell phone, step away from the computer, and allow joy to eclipse routine as your spirit soars. You need to do this especially when you have just experienced a negative emotion, your outlook is wobbling, and you wish to recapture your equilibrium by experiencing three positive emotions. Taking this approach is worth your time; it will change your outlook!

PICTURES OF YOUR MIND

Johnny was born with cerebral palsy. His parents, Joan and Mardian Blair, were advised to place him in an institution—because the Blairs had four other children. Add in Mardian's role as a hospital president, and the consensus was that the couple would be overwhelmed with taking care of Johnny.

But the Blair family chose "the road less traveled" and decided to care for Johnny in their home. They did this for twenty-seven years, during which Johnny never spoke a word and required total care. Johnny's life was compromised physically and mentally, but it was obvious that his spirit was robust—inspired by the loving care of his family.

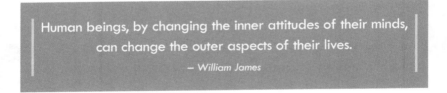

> Human beings, by changing the inner attitudes of their minds, can change the outer aspects of their lives.
>
> — *William James*

I asked the Blairs how they stayed positive given the commitment required to care for Johnny over the years. Joan said, "Sometimes Johnny's situation was discouraging and caring for him was challenging, but the one thing that kept us going was the trust that in heaven Johnny would be made whole and we'd all be together as a family."

I knew that we had to capture this picture to share with other families, and so we asked artist Nathan Greene to illustrate this mental picture in an original painting so that it could inspire other families. Today Greene's picture *Johnny Made Whole* hangs in the Walt Disney Pavilion at Florida Hospital for Children. When we asked showed children a number of religious pictures of artwork hanging in our hospital and asked them to identify their favorite picture in the

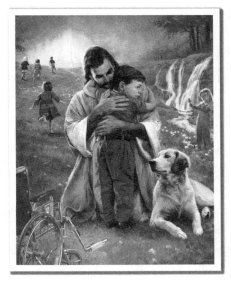

Johnny Made Whole by artist Nathan **Greene**

hospital, they consistently chose this picture over all the rest.

The message of the Blair family is that hope is a journey that contains enough beauty to shine light into gray days and the dark nights of despair. It is all about the picture you remember in your mind and the vision that inspires your spirit.

OUTLOOK CAN BE SHAPED IN THE MORNING

"So let the sun shine in . . . face it with a grin; open up your heart and let the sun shine in . . . ."

These were the words my wife sang to our children each morning as they awoke. Mary Lou is the person in my life who invariably exhibits a positive attitude. Her wake-up ritual began with a morning kiss and a song. She would carry our children in her arms as she opened the window blinds to welcome a new day. I marveled at how they delighted in waking up, smiling and clapping their hands, singing along, and pointing at the creatures they would spot outside. I am not a fan of waking up, but Mary Lou made morning a joy, and I learned how much music can set the outlook for your day. Try it for yourself—choose your own morning song and let music carry you toward a more positive view of life.

THE POWER OF A PROMISE

My father was a self-made optimist. After his family lost their farm and assets in a Canadian drought, they moved to the United States seeking to survive. He was raised during the Depression and drafted into the army to serve in World War II. He had many reasons to be a pessimist, yet despite the negative life experiences he chose to be an optimist. His key? He specialized in a positive mental attitude fueled by promises of hope from Scripture that he had memorized. He had his assistant put them on business-size cards, and he printed sets of them to give to others.

I adopted this practice to lift my spirits during a very difficult period of my life. Mary Lou made them more impactful by copying the promises onto yellow sticky notes and placing them on the mirror in the bathroom and the rearview mirror in my car. It is amazing how a word of inspiration can adjust your outlook. My father taught me to memorize the promises of Scripture as we drove on trips. In those moments we read, discussed, and interpreted into life the promises of God. As a result I learned to live life with optimism, and I am eternally grateful . . . to Dad and to the Lord, who gave him to me.

SCHEDULE AN "INSPIRATION BREAK"

To maintain your positivity ratio, schedule an inspiration break and take a few minutes to allow God to breathe the buoyancy of goodness into you. Actualize one of the following strategies, and watch your positivity soar:

- Recall the goodness that is all around you and give thanks.

- Write a note of affirmation to someone.

- Pause and thank God for his blessings in your life.

- Find a biblical promise and personalize it by putting in your own name.

- Listen to a song or, better yet, sing a song of thanksgiving.

- Take a picture of the beauty that is near you or focus on a piece of fine art that expresses hope to you.

- Enjoy a good laugh—for the joy of the Lord is your strength, and a merry heart is good medicine (see Proverbs 17:22).

If the hurts of life have caused you to become numb to the hope of God, I simply pray that you will sense the breath of heaven filling you with eternal worth, that you may become a living soul. I know it can happen because I have experienced it. I have walked through the valley with friends and family until we could see the light of hope. My prayer for you is that the glasses through which you view life will be milled with the twin lenses of optimism and hope.

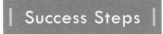

| Success Steps |

- **Borrow Hope When You Need It**: Like Sheila, you will find that the encouragement of others can buoy your own hope, even when it seems like your situation is hopeless.

- **Make Your own Marquee of Hope**: On your mirror, refrigerator, wall, or in some other place that you pass regularly, write positive, optimistic, hopeful words and phrases. Create a sticky pad of hopeful words, and carry it with you for review.

- **Answer Sheila's Husband's Question**: "What are you going to do if you live?" Pretend there is nothing holding you back. How do you want to invest the rest of your life? _____

_____

- **Increase Your Optimism Quotient**: What three things can you do to replace any feelings of pessimism that are dragging you down from optimism?

- **Interpersonal Relationships**: Learn to forgive—don't dwell on the past. Most people want to try to get things to "even" before they will forgive. The truth is, most offenses against us cannot be made right. That's why giving the gift of forgiveness is often the best choice you can make. In the book *Forgive to Live: How Forgiveness Can Save Your Life,* author Dr. Dick Tibbits describes how we are renting space in our head to all manner of painful emotions when we do not forgive. Forgiveness is not admitting someone else is right; it is letting go of being their judge and jury, giving that job to God.

- **Laugh More**: One proponent of the healthy benefits of laughter calls a good belly laugh "inner jogging." He says, "A good belly laugh exercises the diaphragm, contracts the abs, works out the shoulders, leaving muscles more relaxed. It provides a good workout for the heart. Laughing 100 times is equivalent to 10 minutes on a rowing machine, or 15 minutes on an exercise bike."[74] Find and share good jokes, cartoons, and stories that make you laugh. Post them, as appropriate, on your computer and around your house to keep that smile on your face and some levity in your heart.

HEALTHY 100

11

NUTRITION

Feeding the Body, Nurturing the Mind,
Inspiring the Spirit

MOST PEOPLE READING THIS CHAPTER ARE going to expect some diet tips. But in this chapter we want to point out that the most powerful strategy of nutritional health is not only feeding the body but nurturing the mind and inspiring the spirit. Brian's story powerfully illustrates this principle.

TOTAL NUTRITION

The recurring headaches sent the first signals that something wasn't right. Then shortness of breath followed by the twinge of chest pain prompted Brian to swift action. He knew his family history. He had a genetic predisposition for heart disease. His father had quadruple bypass surgery in his early fifties. Brian suspected he might face heart disease at some point in his life, but not at the young age of thirty-nine. It was too early, and he was determined to find the best medical advice available to prevent a repeat of his father's heart history.

Brian's cardiologist confirmed the fears—his heart health was under siege. Lab findings indicated a rare genetic blood disorder had accelerated blockage to critical blood vessels in his heart. The immediate need was to reopen one vessel by implanting a stent. But the threat wasn't over. Within three months Brian needed another stent. And nine months later he required a third stent in the left main descending artery, known as the widow-maker.

Brian and his wife, Tina, had recently expanded their family to five children. This was supposed to be the most productive, robust time of their lives—their prime years. Together they embarked on a commitment to recover full health. They called it "our journey to wholeness" because they believed the key was to design a strategy that inspired the spirit, renewed the mind, and invigorated the body. Heart-healthy nutrition was the most apparent opportunity, but Brian and Tina decided to do more. They pursued a complete CREATION Health makeover. This is the power of Brian's story because instead of simply changing his diet, he pursued a healthy lifestyle. If you are tired of the diet roller coaster, I invite you to embrace the Healthy 100 lifestyle. Brian's story can show you the way:

Unless I took control of what I could do to improve my health, heart disease was going to cut my life short. I would not see my children become adults, fall in love, marry, and raise their families. I knew that I had to rely on physicians to open blocked vessels, but it was up to me to take charge of my health to slow, prevent, and perhaps reverse the blockage.

After my stent procedures I knew I could not simply give in to a genetic reality beyond my control. So I took stock of my lifestyle. Notice I said lifestyle, because I didn't start with diet or exercise. I had to start with priorities. To set my priorities I needed to recalibrate my purpose, so I went back to the personal mission statement I had written years earlier. It became the core around which I shaped my lifestyle. It amazed me how much easier it was to choose the right priorities when my purpose was defined and clear. Two books by Bruce Wilkinson were guides on this journey: The Prayer of Jabez provided inspiration that the Lord would expand my life in His way, and Secrets of the Vine became my textbook for walking with God, free of stress during uncertainty. It was at this time I realized nutrition was more than the food I ate, it included how I fed my spirit and focused my mind.

I set quarterly priorities and shared them with my family and colleagues to develop both support and accountability—support by asking them to understand when I would say yes and when I would turn down requests. Accountability was key in having friends and family hold me responsible for aligning my priorities with my mission. During the first year of lifestyle change, my assistant and I developed a chart to make sure that my daily appointments were in keeping with my priorities. This ensured that my life was re-patterned according to CREATION Health habits.

> While you eat together with family you feast
> on love and laughter.

Next I could control my outlook. The power of a positive outlook was key, and learned optimism was the journey. Practicing optimism is not the natural tendency of the analytical mind of a CFO. This outlook intensified my gratitude for things that I previously took for granted. My greatest joy became evening mealtime as I sat with my wife and children and simply shared the stories of their lives; I listened more intently and heard their hearts as never before.

Following these changes I felt a greater peace, power, and perspective on life. I call it spiritual nutrition. We tend to define nutrition by what we put in our mouths, but I now realize that we are more profoundly impacted by words that come out of our mouths and thoughts that feed our minds. The best way to analyze your nutrition is to review what you are *feeding not only your body, but also your mind and spirit.*

Becoming informed about research in nutrition provided me with the information that focused my mind on the best solutions. My son gave me the book The China Study by T. Colin Campbell that presented convincing evidence of the benefits of a plant-based diet, and I was convinced to pursue a vegetarian diet. This was the first of a series of nutritional changes. The next major change was to adopt strategic eating, which basically means managing energy. My textbook for this change was The Corporate Athlete Advantage by Jim Loehr, PhD.

Eating for energy taught me to manage my blood sugar through healthy snacks at critical times in the day. My heart disease was a drain on my energy, and strategic eating is a significant solution. At work I experienced more consistent focus throughout the day and fewer waves of low energy. Learning the nutritional options for maintaining my blood sugar within an ideal range became key. My mind didn't wonder as much during conversations because I exchanged my coffee breaks for energy breaks. Less caffeine and more protein became my new habit. The impact at home was most noticed by my family. Instead of coming home exhausted and collapsing on the couch, I had enough energy to play with the kids and enjoy the family. I now encourage all of my colleagues and friends to try eating for energy—it has reformed my day.

What are my results to date? For the past few years I simply focused on what I could control in my body, mind, and spirit that influenced my genetic propensity to heart disease. I recently completed the Celebration Health Assessment, Florida Hospital's total health physical program. Every test indicated that I improved over the previous year, and my heart scores, in particular, are showing progress.

What can we learn from Brian's journey to wholeness? Don't settle for a change in diet; go for a lifestyle highlighted by total nutrition. Feed your spirit with mission, feed your mind with the science of nutrition, and feed your body with a plant-based diet.

Perhaps the most powerful aspect of Brian's story is the perspective it brings. The danger of expecting to live longer is that you put off living to your purpose until tomorrow; good intentions pave the path to mediocrity, and you slide into an ordinary life.

THINKING DIFFERENTLY ABOUT FOOD

We are a nation obsessed with food—both with eating it and with not eating it. Television networks and thousands of books are devoted to the topic, and it seems every year there's a new diet that will change our lives. The funny thing is that all the latest and greatest fads usually fall back on some aspect of Eden's original meal plan for man. "Then God said, 'I give you every seed-bearing plant on the face of the whole earth and every tree that has fruit with seed in it. They will be yours for food'" (Gen. 1:29). What did God offer Adam and Eve? Myriad fruits and vegetables, and a wonderful variety of nuts and grains.

I know you won't be surprised to learn that diet was a significant factor in longevity as examined in the book *The Blue Zones*. The Sardinians in Italy consume a lot of omega-3 foods; the Okinawans in Japan eat small portions of low-fat foods; and the Adventists promote vegetarianism.[75]

The advice in the rest of this chapter will tip very strongly toward the non-meat eating lifestyle. I know that doesn't appeal to everyone, but the goal of these CREATION Health principles is to provide you with information practiced by the All-Stars of Longevity that can optimize your quality of life now and increase the likelihood of living a longer, healthier life.

So proceed with an open mind and consider how you might take baby steps toward a plant-based diet, or at least a diet focused on moderate intake of poultry and fish as protein sources. American society has moved far away from this simple diet prescription, but here is the view of Dr. Dean Ornish, whose dietary and lifestyle research has earned widespread popularity among patients and physicians as a way to prevent and reverse cardiovascular disease. "Eating a vegetarian diet, walking (exercising) every day, and meditating is considered radical. Allowing someone to slice your chest open and graft your leg veins in your heart is considered normal and conservative."[76]

> Let food be thy medicine and medicine thy food.
> — *Hippocrates*

Society's focus on food is precisely the problem for most people. Of all the nutritional options available, one is guaranteed to improve your health and enable you to live longer: **eat less**. Dr. Robert Good has conducted research that shows in both animals and humans that if we reduce caloric intake, it will improve just about all aspects of the immune system. In fact, illnesses stemming from an unbalanced immune system become easier to manage. No one is certain of why this happens, although one possible explanation involves a reduction in lifetime exposure to free radicals (toxins that wreak havoc on cells and may contribute to the development of cancer and other diseases).

Whenever you reach a point during a meal when you'd like more, push the plate away and wait ten to fifteen minutes instead of automatically reaching for second or third helpings. If you give your body time to digest, the hunger usually subsides, and you'll be exactly where you need to be in terms of fueling for optimum health.

WHOLE-PLANT FOODS

The influential book *The China Study* by Dr. T. Colin Campbell highlights a comprehensive dietary analysis that began in 1983 and was described by *The New York Times* as "the Grand Prix of epidemiology." It was a collaborative research project by Cornell University, Oxford University, and the Chinese Academy of Preventive Medicine that spanned twenty years. The authors of the study concluded that people who eat a whole-plant food diet that avoids animal proteins and fats from beef, poultry, eggs, fish, and milk will minimize and/or reverse the development of chronic diseases. They also recommended adequate amounts of sunshine to maintain sufficient levels of vitamin D and dietary supplements of vitamin B12 in case of complete avoidance of animal products.

But the benefits of a whole-plant food diet aren't limited to minimizing or reversing chronic disease. According to many experts, such a diet can also help you feel full and lose weight. In the book *The Full Plate Diet*, Drs. Seale, Sherard, and Fleming point out that most whole-plant foods contain a high fiber content. Why is this important? "Dietary fiber makes you feel full. Add fiber to your meals and you'll eat fewer calories. Consume fewer calories than you burn and you'll lose weight . . . Since fruits, vegetables, whole grains, beans, and nuts have lots of fiber and are easy to find, sustainable weight loss is simply a matter of buying healthy foods in the produce section of your grocery store, selecting the best products off the shelf, ordering the right foods on the menu, and not eating unless you are hungry."[77]

With all the concerns about diet today, here's the real bottom line: Keep it simple. Focus on whole-plant foods in as natural a state as possible. I invite you to embrace the CREATION Health principle of nutrition and begin a fresh, balanced relationship with food.

A LASTING GESTURE OF LOVE

We have another very compelling reason to choose a healthy,

balanced diet: in 1960, only 4 percent of American children were considered obese. That number has rocketed past 15 percent. Medical problems that doctors once saw only in adults aged fifty or older are now striking children: heart disease, stroke, high blood pressure, joint problems, and arthritis. And this doesn't include the social and emotional stress children experience when they're overweight.

This is not what we want for our young people. We need to move away from the mindset that sweets and processed foods are treats and a sign of affection. In the book *SuperSized Kids*, Dr. Walt Larimore and nutritionist Sherri Flynt make this basic but important observation, "Children (and most adults) would prefer to make salty, sugary, fatty foods the mainstay of their diets. These foods provide little in the way of nutrition, however, and a lot in the way of calories. Teach your kids that these foods (chips, candy, cookies, etc.) can be enjoyed occasionally (and we stress *occasionally*). Focus instead on foods that provide what the body needs for good health."[78]

BACK TO BASICS

A lasting gesture of love is sharing and teaching kids about the wonderful nutritional basics that God created as a healthy alternative to the salty, sugary, fatty (and fattening) diet just described. And what could be more "basic" than a return to the original "garden" to rediscover God's original design for the human diet—specifically, the daily consumption of a wide variety of whole foods (fruits, vegetables, grains, berries, and grapes)? Studies have clearly demonstrated the difference this one factor makes.

For example, the Adventist Health Study, funded in part by the National Institutes of Health (NIH), focused for thirty years on the life spans of Adventists living in Southern California. The study concluded that strict vegetarians in the group lived, on average, six to nine years longer than the general population.

The study tracked lifestyle factors shown to be statistically significant in predicting longevity, including: regular exercise, a vegetarian diet, smoking history, body weight, and (interestingly) whether they ate a small serving of nuts five to six times a week.

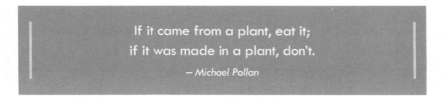

If it came from a plant, eat it;
if it was made in a plant, don't.
— *Michael Pollan*

Demonstrating the effect of lifestyle on longevity (as opposed to simply being an Adventist), the study noted "life expectancy dropped nine to ten years for Adventists who were overweight, past smokers, and non-vegetarian, and who did not exercise or eat nuts regularly."

If you want to increase your chance of one day being called a *centenarian* and enjoy more healthy years of living, then consider the lifestyle factors above as "best practices" to incorporate into your own life. Here is a summary of some discoveries from the first phase of the study:

- Eating nuts several times a week reduces the risk of heart attack by up to 50 percent.

- Eating red meat increases the risk of colon cancer by 60 percent.

- Eating whole-grain bread instead of white bread reduces non-fatal heart attack risk by 45 percent.

- Men who consume a high concentration of tomatoes reduce their risk of prostate cancer by 40 percent.

• Drinking soy milk more than once daily may reduce prostate cancer by 70 percent.

ANOTHER DIMENSION OF LOVE?

God created the human body to run on food, but did you ever wonder why he didn't just come up with some sort of efficient mechanism to get the job done quickly? I'm thinking of tubes we use in the hospital or, since he was capable of anything, one food that contained all the nutrition we need. Eat it in the morning, we're done. But he didn't make us that way.

I think God's design for food and nutrition is a reflection of his nature. He is social, and love is social. So in order to bind us together in another dimension of love, he socialized us around food so we would enjoy the sensory pleasures of eating in the company of others, which enhances that pleasure to a significant degree.

For a moment, let's go deeper than physical reasons for eating well. I believe the key for getting back to the health that God intended is to treat your body with reverence. The apostle Paul said, "Do you not know that your body is the temple of the Holy Spirit who is in you, whom you have from God, and you are not your own? For you were bought at a price; therefore glorify God in your body and in your spirit, which are God's" (1 Cor. 6:19–20, NKJV). This is an extraordinary way of looking at the human body, and yet it is how God views you.

We should eat healthily because we're worth it, because we're called to something noble and great. Our bodies are temples of the Holy Spirit.

WHAT ABOUT WEIGHT?

Of course any discussion of food has to include maintaining healthy body weight. Again, here's one subject Americans can't seem to get enough of. A celebrity gaining or losing ten pounds makes national headlines these days. But let's care for our bodies, not to emulate celebrities, but because our bodies are precious gifts from God—the place where he resides in this world. We want to be as healthy as possible because we want to honor the amazing physical package God created in which to house his Spirit!

If you would like to learn more about how to maintain a healthy body weight, visit our website Healthy100.org for the formula to determine your body mass index (BMI). Measuring your BMI is one of the best ways to determine where you should be. If yours is out of recommended range, it should not surprise you to learn that diet and exercise can turn that around for you.

Remember, you have choice and you have control! And it's not all or nothing. One step at a time is a good start toward a healthier lifestyle.

| Success Steps |

We are bombarded with information and advice about diet and food choices. Make your life easier and look at God's "original" plan for wholeness and balance in body, mind, and spirit.

- **Holistic Nutrition** – In the opening story Brian described the importance of living to your purpose in order to experience an extraordinary life filled with passion and meaning. What is your purpose or mission in life? Does it give you inspiration to live "life to the full" physically, mentally, and spiritually?

- **Eat Fresh** – Include a wide variety of fruits and vegetables in your meals. Try snacking on raw vegetables instead of crackers or chips. Make salads part of your lunch and dinner. When picking your produce, think color—deeply colored vegetables, fruits, herbs, and legumes are packed with disease-fighting plant nutrients and minerals. Buy "organic" when you can, but educate yourself on the benefits of the extra cost, which may vary from one type of produce to another.

- **Nuts and Grains** – Have whole grains at least three times a day—many products are available to choose from. Whole grains are a good source of insoluble fiber, B vitamins, and complex carbohydrates. Don't forget moderate amounts of nuts and seeds, full of soluble healthy fats such as omega-3, omega-6, and vitamin E. They are also excellent sources of protein without cholesterol or the saturated fats found in animal products. Try rice or soy milk on your cereal, and, if you want to go all-out, switch to a soy burger at your next barbecue.

- **Fiber** – In general, the more fiber you eat, the more weight you will lose. When you increase the amount of fiber from whole-plant foods you will have less room for calorie-dense foods.

- **Eat Less** – Think about this. If the nutritional choice to eat less is the single most important life-extending choice anyone can make, what creative ways can you achieve this for yourself and for those you care about? (For example, using smaller plates when you eat at home; saving part of a restaurant portion for later; cutting back or cutting out between-meal snacking; minimizing high-calorie desserts; etc.)

- **Cook From Scratch** – It's almost always healthier to cook from scratch versus reaching for processed or even semi-processed products designed to cut your preparation time. This is because processed food will also most likely cut the basic nutrition delivered while sneaking in some artificial additives or preservatives, or both. When a food label says a product is "enriched," this is usually because the food has been so processed that there is little nutritional benefit left. For example, brown rice has three times more beneficial fiber than fortified white rice, and unlike processed/enriched white flour, healthful wheat germ and bran aren't stripped out of whole-wheat flour.

- **Start Slow** – If you are used to eating meat or are in the habit of consuming higher-fat dairy products, for example, gradually move toward a healthier plan. Make one or two substitutions to start, with a goal of either eliminating red meat entirely or viewing it, as did Thomas Jefferson, as a garnish or part of the "flavor principle."[79] Especially in relation to preparing meals for your family, initiate change slowly and with everyone's knowledge or consent. After all, there is not much future in forcing those whose food you prepare to consume something they may not really like the taste of and that only you are convinced is better for them. Your goal is to instill in them a commitment to better eating and for all the right reasons, since only when that commitment is internalized will it stand the test of the next fast-food temptation.

- **Make It Fun** - Prepared whole foods can look and taste as good as they are for you, but their preparation may take some adjustment on the part of the food preparer. Your local library will have shelves full of cookbooks and meal plans that can inspire you with tasty recipes for meatless dishes. Millions of meatless recipes can be found online to download and enjoy. Your local whole food store will have many suggestions and supplies. Or you might plan a family outing to an area farmers' market to stock up on essentials; the atmosphere is fun, the food is seasonal and fresh, and the prices are usually worth the trip.

12

CREATING YOUR FAMILY'S
HEALTH LEGACY

Passing a Healthy Lifestyle from Generation to Generation

LIFE EXPECTANCY OF OKINAWANS IS DECLIN-ing—the headline shocked me. I read on and found that this celebrated lifestyle which has produced so many of the secrets of longevity is not being passed from generation to generation! Dr. Makoto Suzuki, who coauthored the book *The Okinawa Program*, laments that Okinawan males used to have the highest life expectancy among the Japanese. But this statistic started to decline in the 1990s and was documented in the 2000 Census. Dr. Suzuki and other health experts point out that the younger generation of Okinawans have migrated from the active culture of walking, bicycling, and boating and have embraced riding in a car or bus. This reduction in activity combined with the convenience of fast-food outlets around the US military bases are two causes for the decline of life expectancy and the rise of disease.

This storied culture of health is being eroded —the article goes on to say that one of the most tragic impacts of this change is that the older generation, who continue to practice the health habits of their ancestors, is having to bury their grandchildren. The obvious question is whether the current elders (in their nineties) will be the last generation of Okinawans who live to a healthy 100.

Faced with the demise of Okinawan health and longevity, the question for each of us is how can we inspire our children to adopt a healthy lifestyle? How can we build a health estate that will impact our children and in turn their children, thereby laying the foundation for generations of health?

The good news is that while other lifestyles may be experiencing decline, the Healthy 100 lifestyle continues to increase life expectancy for those who practice it. Establish Healthy 100 goals that motivate each family member despite their age—goals focused on achieving optimal health at each decade of life.

HEALTHY ON THE TENS

The best way to achieve a healthy 100 is to be healthy on the tens. Young children may not be motivated by the goal of a healthy 100— it seems too far off! But being healthy teens, twenties, or thirties is very real, something that can be achieved now. Research the standards of health for each decade and inspire each member of your family to achieve top performance for their age and gender.

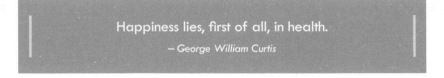

Happiness lies, first of all, in health.
— George William Curtis

The list of All-Stars of Longevity is filled with examples of multigenerational health heroes. The good news is that while other lifestyles may be experiencing decline, the Healthy 100 lifestyle continues to increase life expectancy for those who practice it. In addition, researchers have documented that this lifestyle works in various cultures around the world, despite geography or genetics.[80] Research indicates it is a lifestyle that works in both urban and rural settings.[81] It is also a lifestyle that is transferable across generations. So no matter who you are or where you are, you and your family can benefit from adopting this lifestyle starting today.

This rest of this chapter is a case study of how to pass on a health legacy to your family based on interviewing a family that spans three generations of health. As you read you may be tempted to think, "I should have started this years ago," or, "I wish our family had known about the eight secrets sooner." But wait, this is not about what you, your parents, or grandparents did not do. It is about what you can do now. It is never too late to start. So adopt a healthy future versus regretting an unhealthy past.

To help give you a clearer picture of how this lifestyle can be transferred from generation to generation, let me introduce you to the Houmann family.

Dr. Carl Houmann is a healthy ninety-something; his son Lars is a healthy fifty-something; and his grandson Cameron is a healthy twenty-something. I interviewed each to find answers to how they passed on the eight secrets across three generations. I believe their answers can empower you to inspire a legacy of health for your family.

THE FIRST GENERATION

I arrive at Dr. Houmann's home late in the evening—the flower beds are exploding with color and give evidence to the skill of Anna, a master gardener. She greets me at the front door. This couple is the personification of the All-Stars of Longevity. Since they married in 1948, Anna and Carl have lived through World War II, surviving bombing raids and the German occupation of Denmark. They brought Adventist Health Care to Ethiopia, serving the needs of the royal family and the poverty stricken. But most importantly they shaped a health legacy for their five children.

Carl and Anna met in physical therapy school in Denmark—both were drawn to this profession in order to help others live a more healthy life. This was built into Carl's family heritage—his parents were pioneers of Adventist lifestyle medicine, specializing in physical therapy. Upon their graduation from the School of Physical Therapy the medical director said, "I feel that you should go to Loma Linda in California and study medicine." And before they knew it, Anna and Carl were on their way to America, where Carl completed medical school.

Here are some principles I distilled from my interview with Carl:

- **Think Ageless** – Carl never dwells on his actual age. Subconsciously he thinks he is still in his seventies. He never thinks that he can't do something because he is too old. He just does it.

- **Cherish Sabbath Rest** – Carl and Anna raised their family in a home where the pace of life was often intense. The work responsibilities seemed to consume the week and stress their health. To recover the rhythm of life, they reserved the seventh day of the week for renewal of mind, body, and spirit. Their commitment to an active life in nature played out each Sabbath afternoon. They put aside their daily schedule to enjoy and explore the wonders of God in nature.

  This was also a key to enhancing family communication. Sabbath became the bond around which they built family. Nothing else compares to having undisturbed, uninterrupted time with family—the antithesis of a multitasking lifestyle. Nurturing a commitment to being together as a family and truly becoming friends, and learning how to enjoy each other for who God made each of us to be is central to long-term family love.

- **Start Your Day with God** – Carl spends time in morning meditation and prayer in his garden. This energizes him—renewing his spirit, engaging his mind, activating his body . . . all keys to living long and well.

- **Eat Healthy** – Now in his nineties, Carl believes he never would have reached this age if it hadn't been for the eight health principles. His father and sister both had familial combined type IV hyperlipidemia, and both died prematurely of cholesterol-related heart disease. For this reason Carl adhered to a low-cholesterol, low-fat diet and regularly visited his physician for health maintenance checkups.

- **Live Worry Free** – Carl sleeps well because his motto is: "A sound mind in a sound body." He emphasizes his spiritual life. He believes in God and has peace with him. He has an active prayer life. He meets the challenges of life with the assurance that God is in charge. He doesn't worry about the future; in fact, he looks forward to heaven.

- **Stay Active in Retirement** – Carl and Anna are definitely not couch potatoes. They have hobbies; they exercise. They keep an eye on current events, nationally and internationally. They stay in contact with their professions, they attend meetings, they subscribe to journals, they discuss developments in their fields with former colleagues. They also share common tasks such as housekeeping, shopping, and cooking. The word "retirement" seems to have been removed from their vocabulary.

- **Emphasize Service to Others** – Carl and Anna launched their medical practice in the mission field as a commitment to helping others rather than the more lucrative option of starting a practice near home. This framed his whole family experience because it anchored them in service.

THE SECOND GENERATION

I visited the home of Lars and Julie Houmann two days after they had received the Physicians Pinnacle of Health award from the Celebration Health Assessment (CHA). The CHA physicians grant this award to individuals who score at or above the 80th percentile on the critical measures of health for their age and gender. This is the equivalent of achieving the genius level on an IQ test. It is the first time in the history of CHA that a husband and wife have both achieved this award. They are living at the "Healthy 100 Genius Level." Today the Pinnacle Award is simply another milestone on the journey to a Healthy 100 for Lars and Julie!

As I sat down at the kitchen I asked, "What are your secrets of good health, and what are the keys to passing these on to the next generation?" Here is a summary of their secrets:

- **Make Health Fun** – Strive to live an active life versus a passive life. Try out new things that make being active fun such as hiking, climbing, biking, canoeing, swimming, running, sailing, walking, etc. Cultivate a love for the natural life and learn how to create your own fun in the great outdoors versus having to be entertained by someone or something else.

  Lars and Julie learned to appreciate the wonder of quiet awe in the presence of a mountain vista or the brilliance of stars on a clear night undimmed by the city lights. But above all, they strove to make health fun while also making its pursuit a regular focus. The Houmann family has learned that discipline without joy is drudgery and it seldom transfers to the next generation.

- **Eat Together** — Julie and Lars made a commitment to have the family eat together at least once a day, usually in the evening. It was a struggle to manage schedules, but they made it work. They turned off the TV, silenced the cell phones, and enjoyed a tech-free time focused on family.

- **Nutrition Power** — The Houmanns believe healthy nutrition starts with committing to the best diet at home. Lars dubbed Julie the "bean queen" for her focus on a plant-based diet. Julie points out that she believes food represents the love of the person who made it and that meals should be a celebration of our commitment to each other. Eating right and eating together are hallmarks of health.

- **Reform and Recommit** — Lars and Julie both indicated that during the early years of their family when the children were young and both parents were working they let their health habits drift. But in their late thirties they made a renewed commitment to practicing the eight secrets. Lars became the chief executive officer of Celebration Health, the Florida Hospital facility that was founded on the eight secrets and decided that he needed to model these principles in his own life. For the first time he integrated regular exercise into his daily schedule. Julie's father had had a heart attack at a young age, so she knew that good health practices would be her key to prevention. So she also began a regular fitness routine. No matter what your health history, you can choose today to make better, more consistent choices tomorrow.

- **Embrace A Family Mission** — Ethiopia, the land of Lars' birth, has become a part of the shared family mission that unites the three generations—with all three generations investing their lives in bringing healthcare and learning to this needy country. A few years ago Lars was drawn back to the place where his father practiced medicine. He made a commitment to help strengthen a

Learning Village located outside the capital of Addis Ababa and to open a healthcare clinic at the Learning Village. Lars brought the health education curriculum to life by having the principles of CREATION Health translated into the local language. These principles have become the cornerstone of the school's health curriculum.

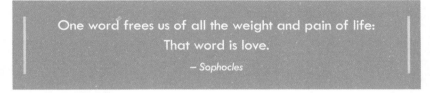

One word frees us of all the weight and pain of life: That word is love.

— *Sophocles*

THE THIRD GENERATION

Cameron, Lars' son and Carl's grandson, is a twenty-something civil engineering student at Walla Walla University in Washington state. As we talk I am listening carefully for his commitment to living the eight principles. I want to know if he thinks they are relevant to his generation or if he considers them to be old fashioned. The first clue comes as I ask Cameron what he considers to be the key to a long and healthy life. His immediate response, "You have to have a sense of purpose and calling that gives you the passion to live life to the full." He's got it—the DNA of the Healthy 100 is not imbedded in the genetics of our children or articulated in the philosophy, it is embodied in the spirit of passion for living that drives the pursuit for optimum health.

The vision of health has passed across three generations in the Houmann family. I am struck by that fact that it has won the minds of the men, because men generally lag behind women in commitment to healthy living. This is evident by the five year life expectancy advantage that American women enjoy over men. At this juncture there is no way to know if Lars and Cameron will achieve Carl's longevity milestones. However, I can tell you they are living healthy on the tens (50's and 20's) and that is the goal. Secondly, I would remind you that the foundation of a Healthy 100 is a passion and purpose for living "life to the full," and it radiates from the language and lifestyle of both son and grandson. We cannot have full control of the number of years we will live, but we can control the intensity with which we will live them.

> The ingredients of health and long life, are great temperance, open air, easy labor, and little care.
> — Sir Philip Sidney

Cameron's health future is bright because he was born into a family who values health, studies it, teaches it, and practices it every day. He has a heritage of health habits that will give life for today and the best opportunity for longevity tomorrow. In talking with Cameron, I gleaned the family health practices that most shaped his life.

- **Environment** – "I was surrounded by health," Cameron said. "My parents and grandparents chose health careers, but more importantly they were committed to teaching health to others. And they lived a healthy lifestyle themselves. My mom set the standards for diet, and my dad set the pace for activity in nature."

- **Activity** – Cameron recalls that his family was very involved in sports personally and in following sports on various levels. His dad is an avid baseball fan, and they often went to games together. Cameron enjoyed team sports such as baseball and basketball, but he also loved the more individual sports of cycling and backpacking, as well as group activities with his family. Playing together as a family kept health fun and bonded them together.

- **Choice** – In Cameron's family they never got accustomed to sitting around with nothing to do. He and his siblings were encouraged to do things that enhanced their lives and taught discipline. One example is music. To excel in music you have to have discipline. You have to focus on theory, practice, and performance. Cameron, his brother Peter, and his sister Kirsten all had music lessons. The friends they made through music had to practice these disciplines as well. All of the kids benefitted from a group of friends who were committed to excellence in music. Music also gave Cameron a positive escape when he became frustrated with life. A practice session would often free him from that frustration, provide enjoyment, and put him back in a good mood.

- **Outlook** – Cameron's greatest sense of satisfaction has come from giving to others in general and to the children of Ethiopia, in particular. This is something he hopes to pass on to future generations. "If kids learn to find happiness through getting they will want more," he said, "but if they learn to find happiness through *giving* they will want to give more. The truth is that giving leads to satisfaction and getting leads only to consumption. Each and every time you give to others it produces a satisfying sense of accomplishment. I returned home determined to engage others in giving, and part of this was joining an already established chapter of Engineers without Borders (a professional group that provides ecologically sensitive and culturally appropriate design assistance to address specific needs in developing countries around the world). My goal is to get more of my colleagues involved in giving versus getting, and in the process we can help a lot of less fortunate folks have a better life."

PASS IT ON

As we learned at the outset of this chapter, the longevity legacy of Okinawa is not universal or assured. Health principles—indeed, life principles—can and must be passed on, generation to generation, as the Houmann family is demonstrating. Now you might be tempted to think that there is something so unique about this family (or their situation) that you could never do the same with your family or in *your* situation. But the Houmann family would respond, "Anyone who really wants to can embrace and practice these principles in their own life or family. It's not easy, but it is simple."

One of our most important callings and opportunities as human beings is to pass on what we have learned about life—including health and faith—to our children. The hope for a healthy future is based on the health of our families. Children of obesity can be replaced by children of opportunity. So why not take this opportunity to plan your Healthy 100 Home!

The financial legacy you or I can pass on to our children may be vastly different from Bill Gates or other billionaires, but we can leave a rich legacy of health. And this is the greatest legacy you can leave for the next generation. You may not be a member of the Fortune 500, but you can be a member of the Healthy 100.

> The greatest wealth is health.
>
> *– Virgil*

13

WHAT INSPIRES YOU TO LIVE?

How Do You Plan to Live as Fully as Possible for as Long as Possible?

I WOULD LIKE TO END THIS BOOK ON A PERSONAL note. I have moved into the grandparent stage of life. As I write this, my wife Mary Lou is flying home from Seattle with our grandchildren Kelsey and DJ. I can't wait for them to arrive so we can launch into a week of making memories that will be another wonderful chapter in our family story. Kelsey and DJ are our living legacy, and I want to inspire them to live "life to the full"—I want them to live CREATION Healthy. To achieve this goal Mary Lou and I have decided we need to model the benefits of CREATION Health in our life so they will want to follow.

GIVE ME THE MOUNTAINS

My first step was to choose a personal biblical text related to aging. It comes from a story in ancient Scripture about a man named Caleb. Caleb was a patriarch of the Israelite people who left the slavery of Egypt behind to travel to the Promised Land of Canaan. After helping conquer the Promised Land it was time for Caleb to choose where he and his family would settle. Eighty-five-year-old Caleb and his friend Joshua were the revered senior citizens of Israel. He could have asked for whatever portion of land that his heart desired. The best of the land lay before him. Yet rather than choose a safe, comfortable piece of land in a conquered territory, Caleb asked for an unconquered, mountainous region populated by giants living in fortified cities. In order to claim this land, he would have to go up and fight for it.

I can imagine that there were people who questioned his judgment. "Why not just retire in a nice green valley and live a quiet life of leisure, fishing by a lake?" they might have asked. But that wasn't Caleb's mindset. "I'll take the mountains!" he said. "And with the Lord's help, we'll drive those giants out" (see Joshua 14).

> Use your imagination not to scare yourself to death but to inspire yourself to life.
> — *Adele Brookman*

He chose the mountains because it was the place of greatest challenge—the stronghold of giants. Caleb knew the land of the greatest threat was also the place of greatest opportunity. It's remarkable that Caleb didn't ask others to go and clear the land for him. He decided to personally lead the quest to settle the most difficult territory in the land. He made a bold statement that implied that he believed he was as strong at eighty-five as he had been at forty-five. What an approach to life!

That is the spirit I want to characterize in my approach to aging. I want to set my eyes on the mountains and challenges of life and not the valleys. I want aging to refine me, not define me. Like Caleb of old, I too want to say, "Give me the mountains!"

In his book *The Blue Zones*, Dan Buettner found that the All-Stars of Longevity don't even have a word for retirement. Instead they focus on *purpose*. That's why this book focuses on achieving health in body, mind, and spirit. It's not enough to strive for physical health alone. Finding and fulfilling your life's purpose is essential because it brings meaning and value to your years.

In fact, the pursuit of purpose is the main reason you're holding this book now. I believe it is part of my life's purpose to share these health principles with you. So I do it through speaking, teaching, and writing. I also seek to apply these principles to my own life. Mary Lou and I are imagining a Healthy 100. This is not a fantasy but a deep desire and a shining hope. Naturally this doesn't guarantee that we will achieve the centenarian milestone, but it does mean we are focused on living each day with our whole body, mind, and spirit—fully alive! We invite you to join us and hope that you will.

WHAT INSPIRES YOU TO LIVE?

If I could sit down and chat with you today, I would ask you to tell me what inspires you to live "life to the full." I would look at the pictures of your family and listen to your stories of life and love. I would hear your heart as you describe the moments where you made memories. I would hear your wisdom about the meaning of life, your hopes for the future of life, and we would share laughter over the humor of life. In short, we would celebrate the joy of living.

After hearing your story, I would ask you one question: how do you plan to live life as fully as possible for as long as possible? Then I would listen to your dreams of health. I'd pull out a pad and together we would design your plan to live CREATION Healthy. As part of that plan, I would tell you that ultimately life is not about living to a hundred—it is about achieving new frontiers of love and meaning that make you want to live to a hundred.

When we finished your plan I would offer to pray for you. My prayer would be simple: *I pray that you may live as long as possible on earth and forever in heaven!*

And now if you'll excuse me, I have grandkids coming, and I have to go and make some preparations for their arrival. We are going to have a blast.

Yours for a Healthy 100,

— Des

ACKNOWLEDGEMENTS

THIS BOOK IS BASED ON THE PREMISE THAT THE model for health is embedded in the Creation story found in the Bible. By applying these eight principles that God built into the Garden of Eden we can experience "optimum vital-ity." My wife, Mary Lou, has helped me to actualize these principles in my life and demonstrate how they can be designed into a care model for the Women's Center at Celebration Health.

My deep appreciation is due to Monica Reed, MD, who implemented these principles as the first medical director of the Women's Center at Celebration Health and continues to promote them now as CEO of Celebration Health. Her insights on this book have been invaluable.

My work at Florida Hospital has been among the most rewarding experiences of my life. I would like to thank Tom Werner and Don Jernigan, PhD, for their unwavering support and encouragement. Without their visionary leadership, Celebration Health and the CREATION Health model wouldn't be what they are today.

Lars Houmann and Brian Paradis have had a lasting impact on my life and helped me to shape many of the ideas in this book. We worked together for more than three years to implement these principles at Celebration Health.

I owe a special debt of thanks to the team who helped create the vision of the CREATION Health principles. My sincere thanks are due to Ted Hamilton, MD, who wrote the original philosophy statement; Dr. Dick Tibbits, who coached the health professionals in implementing it; and Kevin Edgerton, who developed the communications materials to popularize it.

I also want to thank the publishing team who worked so hard to bring this book to life: Todd Chobotar, Dr. David Biebel, Lillian Boyd, Stephanie Lind, and Laurel Dominesey. My thanks are also due to many others who provided valuable feedback as this book took shape including: Eli Kim, MD, George Guthrie, MD, Sy Saliba, PhD, Robyn Edgerton, and Loretta Bacchiocchi, RN.

About the Authors

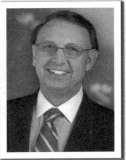

DES CUMMINGS JR., PHD, serves as president of the Florida Hospital Foundation and executive vice president for Florida Hospital, the largest admitting hospital in America. Dr. Cummings holds a PhD degree in leadership and management with emphasis in statistical forecasting. Dr. Cummings also holds a master of divinity degree and is an ordained minister.

Dr. Cummings is committed to promoting health and healing strategies that treat the mind, body, and spirit. Motivated by a vision to help people live to a Healthy 100, Dr. Cummings gave leadership to the development of Celebration Health, a showcase hospital in the Disney city of Celebration, Florida. This facility has attracted national and international attention as a model of health and healing for the twenty-first century.

Dr. Cummings is committed to the concept of empowering patients to take charge of their health and distributing medical knowledge into the community. Dr. Cummings is the author or coauthor of four books including *Creation Health Discovery* (one million in print). He speaks to national and international conferences on the future of healthcare, specializing in strategies for whole person care, healthy communities, and the hospital of the future. It is his belief that we must recreate a new vision of American healthcare for the twenty-first century that is financially viable and enhances quality of life for all Americans. This task calls for the very best thinking of the brightest minds in American healthcare.

In the Cummings home, health and healing is a family affair. Dr. Cummings' wife, Mary Lou, is a nurse and health educator who gave leadership to the development of the Florida Hospital Parish Nurse program and Women's Center at Celebration Health. She has also been an active contributor to the Healthy 100 vision. The Cummings live in Celebration, Florida. They have two adult children, Tracy and Derek, a wonderful son-in-law and daughter-in-law, Denis and Nalani, and two amazing grandchildren, Kelsey and DJ.

MONICA REED, MD, serves as Chief Executive Officer (CEO) of Florida Hospital Celebration Health—a facility recognized by the *Wall Street Journal* as the "Hospital of the Future." As a physician, speaker, author, medical news reporter and hospital administrator, Dr. Reed has dedicated her professional career to promoting health, healing, and wellness. She is also actively involved in hospital development and use of information technology for clinicians in an effort to further enhance patient care.

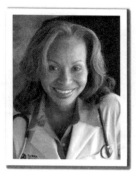

Dr. Reed has filled many other key roles at Florida Hospital in her career, including: senior medical officer—overseeing the relationship between the hospital and its two thousand physicians; medical director for the Celebration Health Center for Women's Medicine; and associate director of the Family Practice Residency Program.

Dr. Reed is the author or coauthor of seven books. She has served as a medical news reporter in Orlando, Florida, and Huntsville, Alabama. In 2008, Dr. Reed was named one of Modern Healthcare's Top 25 Minority Executives in Healthcare.

Dr. Reed is married to Stanton Reed. They have two daughters, Melanie and Megan.

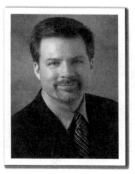

TODD CHOBOTAR serves as founder, publisher, and editor-in-chief of the Florida Hospital publishing program. The focus of his work is creating consumer books, professional monographs, and other resources to help people understand and experience the principles of Whole Person Health. He is the author or coauthor of three books and has served as editor on dozens of publications. Chobotar holds two business degrees from Andrews University. He lives in Orlando with his wife, Jeannine, twins Joshua and Sarah, and two cats Simon & Schuster.

ABOUT THE PUBLISHER

ADVENTIST HEALTH SYSTEM IS A NOT-FOR-profit healthcare organization that emphasizes Christ at the center of care. Founded in 1973 to support and strengthen Seventh-day Adventist healthcare organizations in the Southern and Southwestern regions of the United States, Adventist Health System has grown to become the largest not-for-profit Protestant healthcare provider in the nation.

Today, Adventist Health System supports 43 campuses and employs 55,000 individuals. Adventist Health System hospitals are comprised of 7,700 plus licensed beds, providing care for 4 million patients each year in inpatient, outpatient, and emergency room visits.

In order to best meet the needs of the local communities we serve, Adventist Health System facilities operate independently in hiring employees and delivering care and services. While each entity is unique, they remain united in one mission—*to extend the healing ministry of Christ*. Our mission depends not only on our commitment to Christian ideals but on our efforts to provide nothing less than extraordinary compassionate care.

Adventist Health System's flagship, Florida Hospital, is the largest admitting hospital in America and a national leader in cardiac care. Established in 1908, Florida Hospital now includes almost 2,200 beds on eight campuses. At the turn of the century, the *Wall Street Journal* named Florida Hospital the "Hospital of the Future."

Today, Adventist Health System continues a tradition of whole-person care by adhering to and implementing the CREATION Health model. This is a blueprint for living a healthy and happy life based on the original principles found in the Bible's creation account: **Choice, Rest, Environment, Activity, Trust, Interpersonal, Outlook, and Nutrition.**

Adventist Health System is one portion of the worldwide Seventh-day Adventist healthcare system. To learn more about our hospitals, rehab centers, assisted living centers, nursing homes, and community health programs, all operated within the life-transforming message of Creation Health, please visit these web sites: CreationHealth.com and Healthy100.com.

End Notes

1. Deborah Kotz, "10 Health Habits That Will Help You Live to 100." *US News and World Report*: http://health.usnews.com/health-news/family-health/articles/2009/02/20/10-health-habits-that-will-help-you-live-to-100 (posted February 20, 2009). Accessed 07/05/11.

2. Source: Cystic Fibrosis Foundation, see: http://www.cff.org/AboutCF/Faqs. Accessed 07/05/11.

3. The word "Passionaries" was coined by Barbara Metzler around 2006. For an expansion of this concept, see: www.passionaries.org.

4. D. E. Robinson. *The Story of Our Health Message* (Nashville: Southern Publishing Association, 1965), 146.

5. Howard Markel, MD, PhD, "John Harvey Kellogg and the Pursuit of Wellness," *Journal of the American Medical Association*, May 4, 2011.

6. John W. Rowe, MD, and Robert L. Kahn, PhD. *Successful Aging*. (New York: Pantheon, 1998), 17, 30. Note: This book presents the results of ten years of interdisciplinary research into "successful aging," with one of the authors' main emphases being, "There is increasing evidence that the rate of physical aging is not, as we once believed, determined by genes alone. Lifestyle factors—which can be changed—have powerful influence as well . . . . The bottom line is very clear: with rare exceptions, only about 30 percent of physical aging can be blamed on the genes."

7. Robert Kahn, PhD, "Research Based Lifestyle: Successful Aging Comes to Life." See: http://www.mymasterpieceliving.com/?pageID=47&Research-Based-Lifestyle.html. Accessed 07/05/11.

8. As quoted in: Goodman, Ted. *The Forbes Book of Business Quotations* (New York: Black Dog & Leventhal Publishers, 2007), 285.

9. Grillo M, Long R, Long D, "Habit reversal training for the itch-scratch cycle associated with pruritic skin conditions." *Dermatology Nursing* 19 (3) June 2007: 243-8.

10. For more on this concept I recommend the book entitled, *The Power of a Positive No,* by William Ury (New York: Bantam, 2007).

11. Janet Rae-Dupree, "Can You Become a Creature of New Habits?" *New York Times* (May 4, 2008).

12. Romans 12:21, author paraphrase.

13. Tom Rath, *Vital Friends* (New York: Gallup Press, 2008), 23.

14. Proverbs 24:16, author paraphrase.

15. Dan Buettner, *The Blue Zones* (Washington: National Geographic, 2008), 244.

16. Carol J. Scott, MD. *Optimal Stress* (Hoboken, NJ: Wiley, 2009), 40.

17. Jeannine Aversa, "Poll: Americans stressed out by debt," *Associated Press*, posted on MSNBC.com: http://www.msnbc.msn.com/id/37423674/ns/business-personal_finance/t/poll-americans-stressed-out-debt/. Accessed 07/05/11.

18. "Sleep Habits: More Important Than You Think-Chronic Sleep Deprivation May Harm Health." by Michael J. Breus, PhD (Reviewed by Stuart J. Meyers, MD). See: http://www.webmd.com/sleep-disorders/guide/important-sleep-habits.

19. Sherry Turkle, *Alone Together: Why We Expect More from Technology and Less from Each Other*

(New York: Basic Books, 2011), excerpt posted at: http://www.alonetogetherbook.com/.

20. John Ortberg, "Ruthlessly Eliminate Hurry," *LeadershipJournal.net*. See: http://www.christianitytoday.com/le/currenttrendscolumns/leadershipweekly/cln20704.html. Accessed 07/05/11.

21. Dean Ornish, *Love and Survival: 8 Pathways to Intimacy and Health* (New York: Harper, 1999), Back Cover.

22. See Dan Allerton, *Sabbath-The Ancient Practices* (Nashville: Thomas Nelson, 2010).

23. DeVon Franklin, *Produced by Faith* (New York: Howard Books, 2011), 3.

24. Douglas Cown, Psy.D. Director ADHD Medical Library. See: http://newideas.net/adhd/neurology/reticular-activating-system. Accessed 07/08/11.

25. Ibid.

26. Source: United Nations Population Fund, www.unfpa.org/pds/urbanization.htm. Accessed 07/05/11.

27. *Creation Health Study Guide* (page 72), which also lists the relevant sources. To obtain a copy of *Creation Health Study Guide*, contact Florida Hospital Mission Development at (407) 303-7111, ext. 31, or visit: www.CREATIONhealth.com, and click on "products."

28. See: Ciji Ware, "Declutter Your Life." *AARP The Magazine* (January 2010). Other sources include: http://www.simplifiedinteriors.com/blog/category/clutter-clearing/. Accessed 07/05/11.

29. Evans G, Bullinger M, et al. "Chronic Noise Exposure and Physiology Response: A Prospective Study of Children Living Under Environmental Stress," *American Psychological Society* (January 1998) 9 (1): 75–77.

30. Evans G, Maxwell L. "Chronic noise exposure and reading deficits: The mediating effects of language acquisition" *Environment & Behavior* (September 1997) 29 (5): 638–656.

31. Evans G, Johnson D. "Stress and Open-Office Noise" *Journal of Applied Psychology* (2000) 85 (5): 779–783.

32. Ansel Oliver, "Adventist Burrill, 92, likely sets marathon record," *Adventist News Network*, December 22, 2010.

33. Ibid.

34. Ibid.

35. Ibid.

36. Jeremy Appleton, ND, CNS, "Cut Heart Disease Risk in Half," Healthnotes. As reported at: http://www.bastyrcenter.org/content/view/1121/. Accessed 07/05/11.

37. Dr. John Harvey Kellogg served as the Medical Director for the Western Reform Health Institute—later renamed The Battle Creek Sanitarium. This was the first Adventist healthcare institution and was used as the model for future hospitals and wellness centers. Although Adventist Health System (AHS) did not formally organize until many years after the founding of the Western Reform Health Institute, Dr. John Harvey Kellogg is recognized and honored as the founding medical director of this health system.

38. J.H. Kellogg, *The Living Temple* (Battle Creek, MI: Good Health Publishing Co., 1903), 374.

39. A 2001 study by the Duke University in North Carolina found that exercise is a more effective treatment for depression than antidepressants, with fewer relapses and a higher recovery rate. An earlier Duke study likewise found patients who completed 30 minutes of brisk exercise at least three times a week had a significantly lower incidence of relapse;

only 8 percent of patients in the exercise group had their depression return, while 38 percent of the drug-only group and 31 percent of the exercise-plus-drug group relapsed.

40. Cited by Kristina Fiore, "Four Lifestyle Factors Prevent Cancer, Diabetes, and CVD." (August 10, 2009). See: http://www.medpagetoday.com/PrimaryCare/DietNutrition/15458. Accessed 07/05/11.

41. See: http://www.cdc.gov/speakers/subtopic/speechTopics.html for a discussion of the meaning of the relatively new term, "obesogenic." Accessed 07/05/11.

42. Roger Henderson, MD, Reviewer. "Exercise and heart health." Published at: www.netdoctor.co.uk. See: http://www.netdoctor.co.uk/hearthealth/exercise.htm. Accessed 07/05/11.

43. Paula Span. "Fitness: A Walk to Remember? Study Says Yes." *New York Times* (February 8, 2011). See: http://www.nytimes.com/2011/02/08/health/research/08fitness.html?_r=2, and: http://news.softpedia.com/news/A-Good-Mix-Walking-and-Alzheimer-s-Prevention-169220.shtml.

44. Ron Winslow, "To Double the Odds of Seeing 85: Get a Move On." *Wall Street Journal* (March 9, 2010).

45. See: "Exercise and the Older Adult." ACSM *"Current Comment"* (online posting by the American College of Sports Medicine), at: http://www.acsm.org/AM/Template.cfm?Section=Current_Comments1&Template=/CM/ContentDisplay.cfm&ContentID=8636. Accessed 07/05/11.

46. Monica Reed, MD, *Creation Health Breakthrough: 8 Essentials to Revolutionize your Health Physically, Mentally, and Spiritually* (New York: Center Street/Time Warner Book Group Inc., 2007), 111.

47. Ibid, 113.

48. Ibid, 115.

49. Jeff Levin, PhD, *God, Faith, and Health: Exploring the Spirituality-Healing Connection* (John Wiley & Sons, 2001), 3.

50. *National Geographic* (November 2005).

51. Philip Yancey, *Where is God When It Hurts?* (Grand Rapids: Zondervan, 2002), 183.

52. Linda Hambleton, *If Today is All We Have!* (Orlando: Florida Hospital Publishing, 2011), 186.

53. This story was adapted from the School of Medicine devotional book, Morning Rounds, copyright Loma Linda University, 2008. Used with permission. I am also grateful to Loma Linda University for providing a high resolution photo to include with this story.

54. Stephen Post, *Why Good Things Happen to Good People* (New York: Three Rivers Press, 2008), 1.

55. Ibid, 7.

56. Oman, D., Thoresen, C.E., and McMahon, K. "Volunteerism and Mortality among the Community-Dwelling Elderly." *Journal of Health Psychology* (1999) 4 (3): 301–316.

57. "A Little Volunteering Can Prolong Your Life, U-M Study Finds." *Science Daily*, at: http://www.sciencedaily.com /releases/1999/03/990302150350.htm. Accessed 07/05/11.

58. As quoted by Post, op cit, 2.

59. Tom Rath, *Vital Friends* (New York: Gallup Press, 2008). Kindle version, location 98/1220.

60. As quoted in Rath, op cit. Kindle version, location 172/1220.

61. Blazer, D. "Social Support and mortality in an elderly community population." *American Journal of Epidemiology* (1982) 115 (5): 684–694.

62. Rath, op cit. Kindle version, location 140/1220.

63. Stephanie L. Brown, et al, "Social closeness increases salivary progesterone in humans," *Hormones and Behavior* (June 2009): 108–111.

64. Stephanie Armour, "Friendship and work: A good or bad partnership?" *USA Today* (August 2, 2007). Posted at: http://www.usatoday.com/money/workplace/2007-08-01-work-friends_N.htm.

65. Rath, op cit. Kindle version, location 98/1220.

66. Rath, op cit. Kindle version, location 192/1220.

67. Jerome Groopman, *The Anatomy of Hope* (New York: Random House, 2005), xiv.

68. Davidson, R. J., Kabat-Zinn, J., et al., "Alterations in brain and immune function produced by mindfulness meditation," *Psychosomatic Medicine* (2003) 65: 564–570.

69. Kaplan M, Hugeut N, et al., "Prevalence and Factors Associated with Thriving in Older Adulthood: A Ten-Year Population-Based Study," *The Journals of Gerontology Series A: Biological Sciences and Medical Sciences* (2008) 63: 1097–1104.

70. Musselman D, Evans D, "The Relationship of Depression to Cardiovascular Disease," *Archives of General Psychiatry* (1988) 55 (7): 580–592.

71. Martin Seligman, *Learned Optimism* (New York: Vintage, 2006), 48.

72. Ibid, 4–5.

73. Scott Brady, with William Proctor, *Pain Free for Life* (New York: Center Street, 2006), 49.

74. From the web site of Gerry Hopman, author of *The Power of Humor* (1999): http://www.humor-laughter.com/humor-laughter-health-benefits.html. Accessed 07/05/11. "Inner jogging" was coined by Norman Cousins, author of the classic on the curative power of humor and laughter, *Anatomy of an Illness*. Other citations might include: Sally Beare, *50 Secrets of the World's Longest Living People* (New York: Da Capo Press, 2005), 211-212.

75. See: Dan Buettner, *The Blue Zones: Lessons for Living Longer From the People Who've Lived the Longest* (Washington: National Geographic, 2008).

76. Dean Ornish, as quoted in *Extreme Health: The Nutrition Connection* (Publisher: James A. Guest).

77. Stuart A. Seale, MD, Teresa Sherard, MD, Diana Fleming, PhD, LDN, *The Full Plate Diet: Slim Down, Look Great, Be Healthy!* (Austin, TX: Bard Press, 2009), 10.

78. Walt Larimore, MD, Sherri Flynt, MPH, RD, LD, Steve Halliday, *SuperSized Kids: How to Rescue Your Child from the Obesity Threat* (New York: Center Street/Time Warner Book Group Inc., 2005), 145.

79. Thomas Jefferson, as quoted in *Food Rules: An Eater's Manual*, by Michael Pollan (New York: Penquin, 2009), 54.

80. Tom LeDuc, "The Adventist Contribution to Global Health," part of a larger article entitled "The Adventists and What They Mean to You." on www.WorldLifeExpectancy.com. See: http://www.worldlifeexpectancy.com/what-adventists-mean-to-you. Accessed July 15, 2011.

81. Loma Linda University Adventist Health Sciences Center (2011, June 29). "Black members of Adventist church defy health disparities, study shows." *Science Daily*. See: http://www.sciencedaily.com-/releases/2011/06/110627183946.htm. Accessed July 15, 2011.

Healthy 100 Resources

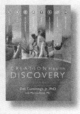

CREATION Health Discovery *(Softcover)*

CREATION Health Discovery takes the 8 essential principles of CREATION Health and melds them together to form the blueprint for the health we yearn for and the life we are intended to live.

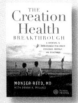

CREATION Health Breakthrough *(Hardcover)*

Blending science and lifestyle recommendations, Monica Reed, MD, prescribes eight essentials that will help reverse harmful health habits and prevent disease. Discover how intentional choices, rest, environment, activity, trust, relationships, outlook, and nutrition can put a person on the road to wellness. Features a three-day total body rejuvenation therapy and four-phase life transformation plan.

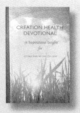

CREATION Health Devotional *(English) (Hardcover)*

Stories change lives. Stories can inspire health and healing. In this devotional you will discover stories about experiencing God's grace in the tough times, God's delight in triumphant times, and God's presence in peaceful times. Based on the eight timeless principles of wellness: Choice, Rest, Environment, Activity, Trust, Interpersonal relationships, Outlook, Nutrition.

CREATION Health Devotional *(Spanish) (Softcover)*

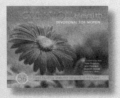

CREATION Health Devotional for Women *(English)*

Written for women by women, the *CREATION Health Devotional for Women* is based on the principles of whole-person wellness represented in CREATION Health. Spirits will be lifted and lives rejuvenated by the message of each unique chapter. This book is ideal for women's prayer groups, to give as a gift, or just to buy for your own edification and encouragement.

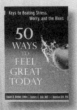

50 Ways to Feel Great Today *(Softcover)*

Feeling a little down? Maybe more than a little down? Here are 50 potential remedies. Changing how we feel often begins with a small thing. Listening to a beautiful song. Enjoying a sunset. Making a happy memory. The book's authors help readers discover how to beat stress, ward off worry, and banish the blues. 50 Ways to Feel Great Today offers medically and scientifically sound advice for giving a blah mood the boot. These time-tested ideas are simple and often low or no cost. While no "be happy" pill exists, the activities in this book equip readers to become their own helping hand.

Healthy 100 Resources

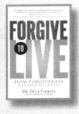

Forgive To Live *(English) (Hardcover)*

In *Forgive to Live* Dr. Tibbits presents the scientifically proven steps for forgiveness – taken from the first clinical study of its kind conducted by Stanford University and Florida Hospital.

Forgive To Live *(Spanish) (Softcover)*

Forgive To Live Workbook *(Softcover)*

This interactive guide will show you how to forgive – insight by insight, step by step – in a workable plan that can effectively reduce your anger, improve your health, and put you in charge of your life again, no matter how deep your hurts.

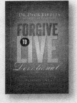

Forgive To Live Devotional *(Hardcover)*

In his powerful new devotional Dr. Dick Tibbits reveals the secret to forgiveness. This compassionate devotional is a stirring look at the true meaning of forgiveness. Each of the 56 spiritual insights includes motivational Scripture, an inspirational prayer, and two thought-provoking questions. The insights are designed to encourage your journey as you begin to *Forgive to Live*.

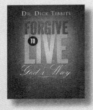

Forgive To Live God's Way *(Softcover)*

Forgiveness is so important that our very lives depend on it. Churches teach us that we should forgive, but how do you actually learn to forgive? In this spiritual workbook noted author, psychologist, and ordained minister Dr. Dick Tibbits takes you step-by-step through an eight-week forgiveness format that is easy to understand and follow.

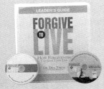

Forgive To Live Leader's Guide

Perfect for your community, church, small group or other settings.

The *Forgive to Live Leader's Guide* Includes:

- 8 Weeks of pre-designed PowerPoint™ presentations.
- Professionally designed customizable marketing materials and group handouts on CD-Rom.
- Training directly from author of *Forgive to Live* Dr. Dick Tibbits across 6 audio CDs.
- Media coverage DVD.
- CD-Rom containing all files in digital format for easy home or professional printing.
- A copy of the first study of its kind conducted by Stanford University and Florida Hospital showing a link between decreased blood pressure and forgiveness.
- Much more!

Healthy 100 Resources

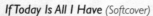

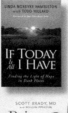

If Today Is All I Have (Softcover)

At its heart, Linda's captivating account chronicles the struggle to reconcile her three dreams of experiencing life as a "normal woman" with the tough realities of her medical condition. Her journey is punctuated with insights that are at times humorous, painful, provocative, and life-affirming.

PAIN FREE FOR LIFE (Hardcover)

In Pain Free For Life, Scott C. Brady, MD, – founder of Florida Hospital's Brady Institute for Health – shares for the first time with the general public his dramatically successful solution for chronic back pain, Fibromyalgia, chronic headaches, Irritable bowel syndrome and other "impossible to cure" pains. Dr. Brady leads pain-racked readers to a pain-free life using powerful mind-body-spirit strategies used at the Brady Institute – where more than 80 percent of his chronic-pain patients have achieved 80-100 percent pain relief within weeks.

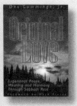

ORIGINAL LOVE (Softcover)

Are you ready for: God's smile to affirm your worth? God's forgiveness to renew your relationship? God's courage to calm your fears? God's gifts to fulfill your dreams? The God who made you is ready to give you all this and so much more! Join Des Cummings Jr., PhD, as he unfolds God's love drama in the life stories of Old Testament heroes. He provides fresh, biblical light on the original day God made for love. His wife, Mary Lou, shares practical, creative ways to experience Sabbath peace, blessings, and joy!

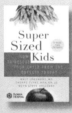

SUPERSIZED KIDS (Hardcover)

In SuperSized Kids, Walt Larimore, MD, and Sherri Flynt, MPH, RD, LD, show how the mushrooming childhood obesity epidemic is destroying children's lives, draining family resources, and pushing America dangerously close to a total healthcare collapse – while also explaining, step by step, how parents can work to avert the coming crisis by taking control of the weight challenges facing every member of their family.

SUPERFIT FAMILY CHALLENGE - LEADER'S GUIDE
Perfect for your community, church, small group or other settings.

The *SuperFit Family Challenge Leader's Guide* Includes:

- 8 Weeks of pre-designed PowerPoint™ presentations.
- Professionally designed marketing materials and group handouts from direct mailers to reading guides.
- Training directly from Author Sherri Flynt, MPH, RD, LD, across 6 audio CDs.
- Media coverage and FAQ on DVD.
- Much more!

"Come near to God and he will come near to you..." – James 4:8, NIV

www.FloridaHospitalPublishing.com

 www.Facebook.com/FloridaHospitalPublishing

LEAD YOUR COMMUNITY
TO HEALTHY
LIVING

With C·R·E·A·T·I·O·N Health
Seminars, Books, & Resources

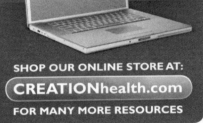

SHOP OUR ONLINE STORE AT:

CREATIONhealth.com

FOR MANY MORE RESOURCES

SEMINAR MATERIALS

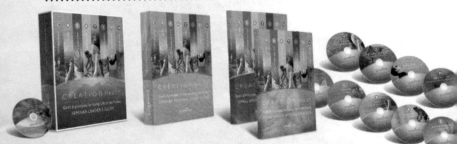

Leader Guide
Everything a leader needs to conduct this seminar successfully, including key questions to facilitate group discussion and PowerPoint presentations for each of the eight principles.

Participant Guide
A study guide with essential information from each of the eight lessons along with outlines, self assessments, and questions for people to fill-in as they follow along.

Small Group Kit
It's easy to lead a small group using the CREATION Health videos, the Small Group Leaders Guide and the Small Group Discussion Guide.

GUIDES AND ASSESSMENTS

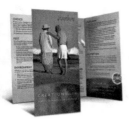
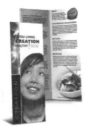
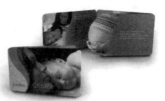

Senior Guide
Share the CREATION Health principles with seniors and help them be healthier and happier as they live life to the fullest.

Self-Assessment
This instrument raises awareness about how CREATION Healthy a person is in each of the eight major areas of wellness.

Pregnancy Guides
Expert advice on how to be CREATION Healthy while expecting.

Pocket Guide
A tool for keeping people committed to living all of the CREATION Health principles daily.

GET ORGANIZED!

Tote Bag
A convenient way for bringing CREATION Health materials to and from class.

Presentation Folder
Keep CREATION Health notes and resources organized and in one place.

MARKETING MATERIALS

Postcards, Posters, Stationary, and more
You can effectively advertise and generate community excitement about your CREATION Health seminar with a wide range of available marketing materials such as enticing postcards, flyers, posters, and more.

CREATION HEALTH BOOKS

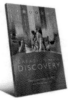

CREATION Health Discovery
Written by Des Cummings, Jr., PhD and Monica Reed, MD, this wonderful companion resource introduces people to the CREATION Health philosophy and lifestyle.

The CREATION Health Breakthrough
Written by Monica Reed, MD, this book guides you through a personal weekend retreat that will integrate healthy behaviors into your lifestyle and rejuvenate your life.

Did You Enjoy This Book?

Why not get copies for your family, friends, business, church, community or small group study?

8 Secrets of a Healthy 100 is available at discounted rates if you order in quantity.